TROPICAL DISEASES - ETIOLOGY, PATHOGENESIS AND TREATMENTS

CHIKUNGUNYA

EPIDEMIOLOGY, TRANSMISSION AND THERAPEUTICS

TROPICAL DISEASES - ETIOLOGY, PATHOGENESIS AND TREATMENTS

Additional books and e-books in this series can be found on Nova's website under the Series tab.

TROPICAL DISEASES - ETIOLOGY, PATHOGENESIS AND TREATMENTS

CHIKUNGUNYA

EPIDEMIOLOGY, TRANSMISSION AND THERAPEUTICS

PHILLIP GALVAN
EDITOR

nova
Medicine & Health
New York

NOTICE TO THE READER

Library of Congress Cataloging-in-Publication Data

ISBN: 978-1-53619-978-9

Published by Nova Science Publishers, Inc. † New York

CONTENTS

PREFACE

Chikungunya (CHIKV) is a viral infection spread by mosquitoes that can cause symptoms such as fever, joint pain, muscle pain, headache, fatigue, and rash, which can become severe. While symptoms generally subside within a week or two, the disease nonetheless imposes a burden on societies around the world and carries a death risk of 1 in 1,000 infections. Chapter One details the history and evolution of the virus, including its epidemiology and extensive spread, and discusses disease prevention and vector control measures. Chapter Two describes the geographical distribution, transmission, and alternative hosts of Chikungunya. Chapter Three provides an insight into the different immunotherapy and immunoprophylaxis strategies that have demonstrated promising results so far for the treatment of this disease. Lastly, Chapter Four provides an overview of the potential therapeutics that have been proposed and developed for CHIKV.

Chapter 1 - Chikungunya is a deadly mosquito-borne disease that is endemic in Asia and Africa. Like all alphaviruses, the Chikungunya virus has a spherical shape and lipid envelope, with spiked structures of glycoprotein trimers on the surface to attach to host cells. It is around 70 nm in diameter and contains approximately 11.8kb of single-stranded positive sense RNA genome. Transmitted via mosquito bites, the onset of illness can range up to 12 days, where common symptoms include prolonged high fever and severe joint pains, with a death risk of 1 in 1,000. The Chikungunya virus was first detected in Tanzania in 1952. Although infections have died down in the 1970s, in the 2000s, large outbreaks were reported in Africa,

Asia, Europe, India and the Pacific Ocean nations. The virus was reported in Caribbean countries for the first time in 2014, and since then, it has spread throughout America. There is neither a vaccine for the virus, nor a specific medication to treat its infection. As such, the Chikungunya virus has become a prevalent threat. This chapter details the history and evolution of the virus, including its extensive spread, epidemiology, and the burden it incurs on countries and their citizens. Disease prevention and vector control measures are also briefly discussed.

Chapter 2 - Chikungunya is a re-emerging acute febrile illness whose outbreaks have been documented globally. Chikungunya outbreaks have occurred in several continents and countries with the first Chikungunya virus being isolated from the serum of a febrile patient in Tanzania in 1953. From 1953 several suspected and laboratory confirmed cases have been reported in East Africa, Indian Ocean Islands, Asia, Europe, North America and the Caribbean Islands. During these outbreaks, some fatalities associated with this outbreaks have been documented like in Reunion Island outbreak of 2005. The spread of Chikungunya virus in a number countries occurred due to the arrival of Chikungunya infected travelers from endemic countries, for example, India and Europe received infected travelers from the Indian Ocean Islands. As recent as 2020, Chikungunya outbreaks are still being reported. The distribution of Chikungunya has been associated with new vectors that can competitively transmit this virus. Chikungunya virus transmission occurs in two cycles: sylvatic and urban cycle. In Africa, the virus is maintained in a sylvatic cycle which includes non-human primates (chimpanzees, monkeys and baboons) and different species of mosquitoes that dwell in the forests. Chikungunya virus may have evolved from these forest-dwelling mosquitoes in Central Africa, and then adapted to an urban cycle as it spread from Africa through the Indian Ocean Islands, then to Asia. In the urban cycle which has been reported in Asia and urban settings, the virus is transmitted via *Aedes aegypti and Aedes albopictus* mosquitoes to human through the bite of an infected mosquito. Transmission and spread of Chikungunya and other viral diseases should be closely monitored by performing routine surveillance to prevent economic losses that may come with disease outbreaks.

Chapter 3 - The resurging CHIKV outbreaks and epidemics have presented several socio-economic challenges to the world. Even after 60 years of its discovery, there are still no approved therapies or vaccines. The scientific community today is in pursuit of rapid development of antivirals and prophylactics. In this chapter, the authors provide an insight into the different Immunotherapy and Immunoprophylaxis strategies that have demonstrated promising results so far and are under development and others that are developed and approved for CHIKV.

Chapter 4 - Since its first presence in Tanzania in 1952, the Chikungunya virus (CHIKV) has caused several severe outbreaks and epidemics throughout the world, affecting nearly 40 countries. This arthropod-borne virus is responsible for causing musculoskeletal inflammatory disease in humans. With rising global temperatures, that encourage the growth of the *Aedes* mosquito and lack of approved therapeutics, the risk of future outbreaks expanding beyond the confines of the tropics has significantly increased. As of now, there are no FDA-approved therapeutics available for the treatment of chikungunya however, many are in pipeline and are awaiting clinical trials. The recurring and sporadic CHIKV outbreaks and epidemics mandate the need for potent therapeutics against the virus. In this chapter, the authors intend to provide an overview of the potential therapeutics that have been proposed and developed for CHIKV.

In: Chikungunya
Editor: Phillip Galvan
ISBN: 978-1-53619-978-9

Chapter 1

Chikungunya Virus: History, Evolution, Current Epidemiology and Its Burden to the World

***Neevaarthana Subramaniam*[2] *and Nor Fazila Che Mat*[1,*]**
[1]Biomedicine Program, School of Health Sciences,
Universiti Sains Malaysia, Kubang Kerian. Kelantan, Malaysia
[2]Environmental and Occupational Health Program,
School of Health Sciences, Universiti Sains Malaysia,
Kubang Kerian, Kelantan, Malaysia

Abstract

Chikungunya is a deadly mosquito-borne disease that is endemic in Asia and Africa. Like all alphaviruses, the Chikungunya virus has a spherical shape and lipid envelope, with spiked structures of glycoprotein trimers on the surface to attach to host cells. It is around 70 nm in diameter and contains approximately 11.8kb of single-stranded positive sense RNA

* Corresponding Author's E-mail: fazilacm@usm.my.

genome. Transmitted via mosquito bites, the onset of illness can range up to 12 days, where common symptoms include prolonged high fever and severe joint pains, with a death risk of 1 in 1,000. The Chikungunya virus was first detected in Tanzania in 1952. Although infections have died down in the 1970s, in the 2000s, large outbreaks were reported in Africa, Asia, Europe, India and the Pacific Ocean nations. The virus was reported in Caribbean countries for the first time in 2014, and since then, it has spread throughout America. There is neither a vaccine for the virus, nor a specific medication to treat its infection. As such, the Chikungunya virus has become a prevalent threat. This chapter details the history and evolution of the virus, including its extensive spread, epidemiology, and the burden it incurs on countries and their citizens. Disease prevention and vector control measures are also briefly discussed.

INTRODUCTION

Chikungunya is a disease caused by the Chikungunya virus (CHIKV). Due to the similarity of symptoms, it is often misdiagnosed as dengue in the early stages of infection. However, researchers have discovered that this virus is different than the flavivirus that causes dengue, although they the *Aedes* mosquito as a common vector. Since then, CHIKV has become prevalent in many countries around the world. Several control measures have been developed to curb its spread along with dengue virus (DENV). Although the number of cases and deaths caused by CHIKV is far fewer than DENV, the former disease is still considered a menace as it has the same virulence and capability to spread and infect people like the latter.

This chapter aims to inform readers about the history and early transmissions of CHIKV, the extensive outbreaks that happened after that, its current epidemiology, and how the disease has burdened the economy of endemic countries, besides the prevention measures taken by health authorities worldwide. All the topics are interesting and important to discuss, considering the fact that CHIKV infection is a phenomenon that can be related to the ability of the virus to re-emerge and form new transmissions in a particular country.

CHIKV also poses a challenge to the public healthcare system in many countries. There is no medication to treat the virus, and treatment is mostly applied to relive symptoms. Meanwhile, the development of vaccine is taking an extremely long time to be available as the disease is not considered a serious global threat compared with SARS-CoV-2, which causes Covid-19. The urgency of a pandemic has led to multiple vaccines being developed against Covid-19, using all sorts of technology (encapsulated mRNA, viral vectors, nanoparticles and attenuated viruses), with most of them receiving World Health Organization (WHO) approval in less than two years. As for Chikungunya, even though it has been declared a pandemic by WHO, it has fallen into one of the neglected tropical diseases due to its sporadic nature and low urgency, which also makes it unattractive for the pharmaceutical industry to find a cure. Now, preventive measures like awareness campaigns and controlling the population of *Aedes* mosquitoes is the only way to keep CHIKV at bay.

History of CHIKV Transmission

The CHIKV is an alphavirus that belongs to the Togaviridae family that is, transmitted among humans through *Aedes* mosquito bites (Griffin 2013). The name Chikungunya is derived from, the Makonde language in southeast Tanzania, Africa, where the disease was first described in 1952. The Makonde root verb is *kungunyala*, meaning 'that which bends up,' 'to become contorted' or 'to walk bent over' (Gudo et al. 2016). The disease is described so because it causes patients to suffer 'bent' joints, which is reflected by their stooped posture and severe pain and swelling in the wrists, hands, ankles and knees (Bonthius 2012; World Health Organization 2021). Besides joint pains and swelling, other main symptoms include prolonged high fever, followed by nausea, fatigue, headaches and rashes (World Health Organization 2020). High-risk groups include people above age 65 and neonates (Staples et al. 2020). Elderly people with chronic health problems are likely to develop long-term complications such as rheumatological disease (Staples et al. 2020). Neonates are susceptible as the virus may be transmitted from mother to baby, and due to their under-developed immune system, their mortality rate is higher (Staples et al. 2020).

Research on the virus phylogeny revealed that CHIKV has four lineages (Galan-Huerta et al. 2015). The first phylogenetic study reported that the virus originated from Africa with two major lineages, the West African and the East/Central/South African (ECSA) genotypes (Galan-Huerta et al. 2015). It was also discovered that the ESCA lineage had spread to Asia, giving rise to a third lineage, known as the Asian genotype (Volk et al. 2010). The fourth lineage was reported much later after an outbreak in Kenya in 2003, where the virus had similarities with the ESCA genotype and another virus originating from Indian Ocean countries (de Lamballerie et al. 2008; Galan-Huerta et al. 2015).

CHIKV infection was first described in the 1950s, where it was initially observed to be transmitted among non-human primates through the in a sylvatic cycle (Weinbren et al. 1958). Subsequently, the first virus spread to humans was identified in a patient with febrile illness during a dengue epidemic in Tanganyika (present day Tanzania) between 1952 and 1953 (Mason and Haddow 1957). The febrile illness was recognised as a symptom distinct from dengue, and the disease was named Chikungunya. Chikungunya may be diagnosed on the basis of clinical, epidemiological and laboratory techniques. Based on clinical presentation alone, it is very difficult to differentiate between DENV and CHIKV infection, however, in CHIKV infection, joint pains are much more prominent and can be used as a distinguishing feature (Shiferaw et al. 2015). And unlike dengue, Chikungunya also does not cause haemorrhagic complications. Epidemiological data includes the patient's travel history to pandemic places within the last 12 days, which is the virus' incubation period. Laboratory techniques include decreased lymphocyte count. Specific tests like viral isolation, serological testing (enzyme-linked immunoassay) and reverse-transcription PCR will provide definitive results, but they require as the tests must be conducted under level 3 biosafety protocols (Johnson et al. 2016).

The clinical and epidemiological characteristics of CHIKV were first described by Marion Robinson and W. H. R. Lumsden in 1955 (Shiferaw et al. 2015). In the early years, the geographical distribution of CHIKV was first identified in east Africa, specifically at the Makonde Plateau of Tanzania, near the border with Mozambique (Zeller et al. 2016; Sowards

2019). Soon after, the virus began spreading throughout the sub-Saharan part of the continent, with sporadic outbreaks occurring in South Africa, Zimbabwe, the Democratic Republic of Congo, Zambia, Senegal, Uganda, Nigeria, Angola, and the Central African Republic up to the late 1970s. The historical timeline of CHIKV spread in Africa in shown in Figure 1 (Jupp and McIntosh 1988; Powers and Logue 2007; Desdouits et al. 2015; Zeller et al. 2016).

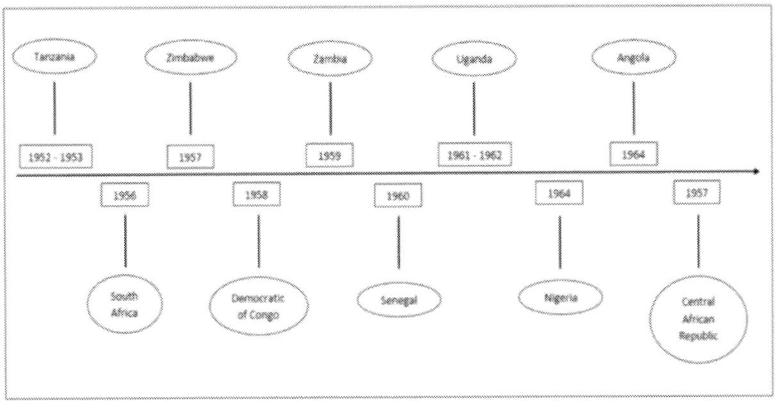

Figure 1. History timeline and spread of Chikungunya outbreaks in Africa since 1952.

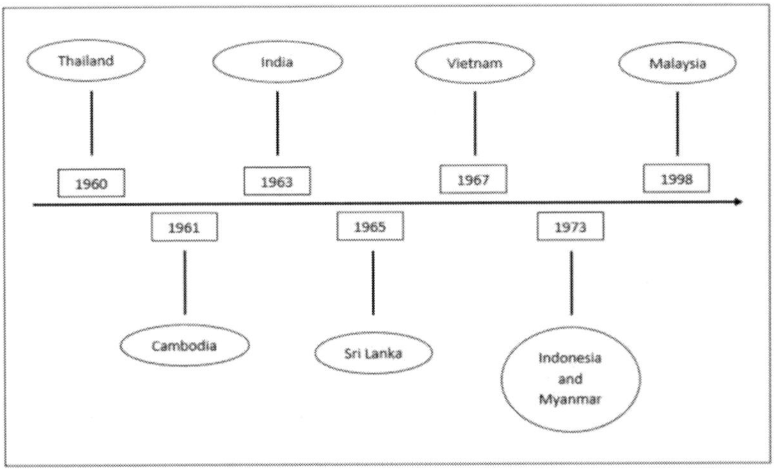

Figure 2. History timeline and spread of Chikungunya outbreaks in Asia since 1960.

Whereas in Asia, the virus was first detected in Bangkok, Thailand, in 1960, which then spread to Cambodia, India, Sri Lanka, Vietnam, Indonesia, Myanmar and Malaysia until the 1990s as shown in the historical timeline in Figure 2 (Chastel 1963; Deller and Russell 1967; Mendis 1967; Thaung et al. 1975; Zeller et al. 2016; Harapan et al. 2019). Although the virus has spread to almost all major countries in Asia in the 1990s, these countries, however, only reported a low number of cases. Outbreaks are sporadic and only occurs occasionally after 1973 (Zeller et al. 2016; World Health Organization 2020). This has caused Chikungunya to fall into a group of neglected tropical diseases.

EXTENSIVE TRANSMISSION AND GEOGRPHICAL DISTRIBUTION OF CHIKV ACROSS THE GLOBE

CHIKV has spread to many areas of the world and the disease is showing a mostly re-emerging trend. The spread of CHIKV is caused by the prevalence of *Aedes* mosquitoes and human activities, such as travelling and trade (Wahid et al. 2017). The CHIKV epidemiological pattern is known to be sporadic and endemic in several parts of Africa (Wahid et al. 2017). After all the initial occurrences, intermittent major outbreaks have occurred for the next seven to 20 years (Pialoux et al. 2007). Although the mortality rate had been relatively low, CHIKV still poses a threat to public health, causing an increased burden in the healthcare system of affected countries.

Transmission of CHIKV

The CHIKV is carried by two specific female Aedes lineages – the African and Asian lineages. Species like Aedes furcifer, *Aedes luteocephalus*, and *Aedes taylori* are the main vectors in West Africa, while *A. furcifer* and *Aedes cordellieri* carry the disease in other parts of the continent (Grandadam et al. 2011). In Asia, disease transmission is facilitated by *A. aegypti* and *A. albopictus* (Grandadam et al. 2011). *A. aegypti* is usually found in the tropics while *A. albopictus* is mostly limited to temperate regions (Sanyaolu et al. 2016). However, as an invasive species itself, *A. albopictus (*which is native to Asia*)* has been reportedly found in Africa, America and Europe (World Health Organization 2020). The female mosquitoes feed on blood during the day, especially in early mornings and late evenings (Sanyaolu et al. 2016; World Health Organization 2020*)*. Outbreaks of Chikungunya is observed to occur every three to four years (Vega-Rua et al. 2015; Sanyaolu et al. 2016). Transmission is also reported to be temperature dependent, effecting the virulence of CHIKV in Aedes mosquitoes (Diallo et al. 1999). Few years ago, the CHIKV was identified as a category C priority pathogen, where rhis classification means the virus has a potential to become a biological weapon and should be handled under level 3 biosafety conditions (Glushakova et al. 2017).

Two types of transmission cycles have been identified in the spread of CHIKV. The first is the enzootic or sylvatic transmission cycle. This cycle was responsible for the first few outbreaks in rural areas (Simon et al. 2011). It usually occurs among wild animals in forests, where *Aedes* mosquitoes populate (Galan – Huerta et al. 2015). In the forest areas, non-human primates, such as monkeys and other mammals like bats and squirrels serve as reservoir and hosts that amplify the virus (Matusali et al. 2019). This cycle is uncontrollable as it is difficult to track when and how the virus transmits among wild animals (Figueiredo 2019). As such, this transmission cycle that only involves forest animals in the beginning stages may have spilled over to rural communities, where humans become the incidental or dead-end hosts (Galan – Huerta et al. 2015).

The second type of transmission cycle is the urban cycle, which occurs between *Aedes* mosquitoes as vectors, and dense human populations as the hosts (Galan – Huerta et al. 2015). *Aedes* mosquitoes seem to be the main vectors in both cycles because they can be both zoophilic and anthropophilic (attracted to humans and animals as a source of food) (Crawford et al. 2017). This cycle is also known as the endemic or epidemic cycle (Valentine et al. 2019). The urban cycle increases human exposure to the disease as mosquitoes are capable of inhabiting human residential areas and surviving among human populations (Galan – Huerta et al. 2015). It has been observed that during inter-epidemic periods, animals act as CHIKV reservoirs while in large outbreaks, humans become the main reservoirs (Gobbi et al. 2015). This epidemic transmission is possible because female mosquitoes prefer humans as their bloodmeal since they can lay eggs in man-made containers and live inside the houses of human hosts (Weaver et al. 2012). In addition, a previous research suggested that *A. albopictus* populations have spread all over the world through the export of timber from Asia (Reiter and Sprenger 1987). These factors not only lead to successful urban adaptation of *Aedes* mosquitoes, but also contributed to a large-scale spread of CHIKV. This cycle is, however, also reversible and the virus is able to jump back to sylvatic maintenance cycles among wild animals (Figueiredo 2019).

Global Expansion and Geographical Distribution

After years of sporadic infections in most countries, a large Chikungunya outbreak of about 13,500 cases occurred in Lamu Island, Kenya in July 2004 (Sergon et al. 2004). The disease then spread to the island nation of Comoros and the French overseas territory of La Reunion in the Indian Ocean, where 35% of the latter island's population were infected in 2005 (Pialoux et al. 2007; Renault et al. 2007). The La Reunion epidemic produced unfamiliar clinical complications in its victims, where 123 cases were reported with severe symptoms (Renault et al. 2007). In the same year, India also reported several outbreaks, which were likely due to CHIKV co-infection with DENV in the states of Andhra Pradesh, Orissa and Maharashtra (Collao et al. 2010; Saswat et al. 2015). Vertical transmission and neurological manifestations were observed among children in La Reunion and India (Mohamat et al. 2020). When the disease was confirmed, the year marked the first large-scale return of Chikungunya in India since the 1970s, which went on to infect more than 1.3 million people in 13 states (Arankalle et al. 2007).

The increase of outbreaks in India then triggered the re-emergence of Chikungunya in Indian Ocean islands and countries, as well as Southeast

Asia in 2007 (World Health Organization 2006; Powers and Logue 2007). These include Sri Lanka, Maldives, Malaysia, Indonesia, Philippines and Thailand (Rezza et al. 2007). Even Europe was not spared when cases were reported in the north-eastern parts of Italy (Rezza et al. 2007). In Indonesia, Chikungunya cases were reported as a mild and short illness, occurring during the dry season with a low incidence (Laras et al. 2005; Kosasih et al. 2013; Zeller et al. 2016). In Malaysia, the disease re-emerged in Perak after a lull of seven years, when a traveller from India brought the virus into the country (Zeller et al. 2016). Since then, cases had been continuously rising. In 2009, infections were recorded again in La Reunion and this time, the virus had spread to Europe, the United States (USA), Singapore and Taiwan in 2010 (D'Ortenzio et al. 2011; World Health Organization 2020). CHIKV infection during that period was facilitated by travel boom, thanks to a recovering world economy and globalisation (World Health Organization 2020). During the period, this disease was declared an epidemic by the World Health Organization.

The geographical spread of the invasive *A. albopictus* was considered the main reason in the increase of Chikungunya cases worldwide (Paupy et al. 2012). In fact, between 2005 and 2009, major cities in Central and West Africa had large populations of *A. albopictus*, especially in Cameroon, Libreville and Gabon (Zeller et al. 2016). The same problem was also reported in the city of Montpellier in Southern France (Vega-Rua et al. 2013; Zeller et al. 2016).

From 2011 to 2013, major transmissions of CHIKV were observed in Western and Central Africa, Oceania, Europe, South Asia, South-east Asia and Western Indian Ocean Islands (Caglioti et al. 2013). In the Pacific region, Chikungunya was detected in New Caledonia in early 2011 and had spread to Yap State in Micronesia in 2013 (Aubry et al. 2015). In Africa, an outbreak in Brazzaville, Republic of the Congo, affected 8,000 people until the locals dubbed the disease 'robot malaria' due to impairments in the victims' posture and movement (Mombouli et al. 2013). In Southeast Asia, Chikungunya had been reported in major cities like Manila, Singapore and Jakarta (Zeller et al. 2016).

Chikungunya arrived in China, Cambodia, Papua New Guinea and Bhutan between 2010 and 2012, where the infections involved a mutant genotype of the ECSA virus lineage (Qiaoli et al. 2012; Sam et al. 2012; Saswat et al. 2015; Zeller et al. 2016). In 2014, autochthonous CHIKV infections were reported for the first time in the American mainland, starting from El Salvador in June 2014, before making their way north to USA, and south to Costa Rica, Panama and Venezuela in the following month (Pan American Health Organization 2014a; Pan American Health Organization 2014b). These autochthonous infections first arrived through the Caribbean Island of Saint Martin in early 2014, before spreading to neighbouring islands and the American island (Bortel et al. 2014; Leparc-Goffart et al. 2014). By the end of the year, Chikungunya large part of central and south America, including Mexico, Belize and Honduras (Pan American Health Organization 2014c; Galan-Huerta et al. 2015).

Simultaneously, the United Kingdom and France recorded the highest number of cases in (World Health Organization 2020). A CHIKV-DENV coinfection was also reported in Portugal, which was brought in by a traveller from Angola (Parreira et al. 2014). CHIKV infections recorded in Pacific Islands such as Tonga, American Samoa, the Independent States of Samoa and Tokelau were believed to originate from the same Asian genotype as well (Aubry et al. 2015; Zeller et al. 2016). Meanwhile, CHIKV infections in French Polynesia was apparently introduced from the Caribbean (Aubry et al. 2015). In 2015, a smaller number of CHIKV cases were recorded compared to 2014, however, the virus had resurfaced in Senegal, Africa after five years (Diop et al. 2015; World Health Organization 2020). South American nations recorded the highest number of Chikungunya cases in 2015, with Colombia contributing the highest number (World Health Organization 2020).

In 2016, outbreaks seemed to peak in Brazil, Bolivia and Colombia (World Health Organization 2020). The very same year, an autochthonous transmission of CHIKV was detected in Argentina for the first time after an outbreak of 1,000 cases (World Health Organization 2016). Major outbreaks were also observed in Kenya, Somalia and India, while European countries reported fewer than 500 cases only (World Health Organization 2020).

Progressing to 2017, the European countries recorded a slight increase in the number of cases, with Italy contributing the most from August to October (European Centre for Disease Prevention and Control 2017; World Health Organization 2020). New autochthonous CHIKV infections were also detected in France and Italy for the first time since 2014 (World Health Organization 2020).

On the whole, regardless of the countless number of efforts taken to contain Chikungunya, new infections always appeared, creating sporadic epidemics everywhere. South Asia and South America were the most affected regions, where many cases were reported in India, Pakistan, the Caribbean nations and Brazil (World Health Organization 2020). CHIKV is still actively circulating worldwide, with new outbreaks detected in Sudan, Yemen, Cambodia and Chad from 2018 to 2020 (World Health Organization 2020). This shows that CHIKV is a persistent virus that causes a burden to developing countries on top of other infectious diseases.

Current Epidemiology on CHIKV

CHIKV is endemic in several continents, including Africa, Asia and in sub-tropical regions of America (European Centre for Disease Prevention and Control 2021). In contrast, Europe and the Pacific region are not reporting on any newer Chikungunya cases to date (European Centre for Disease Prevention and Control 2021). A recent study found that CHIKV is the second most problematic arbovirus after DENV (James et al. 2018; Puntasecca et al. 2021). In fact, a review on CHIKV cases between 2009 and 2019 states that there may have been inconsistencies in the reporting of CHIKV cases, especially in areas without proper screening and surveillance, resulting in a fewer number of cases being reported (Puntasecca et al. 2021). The current prevalence and epidemiology of CHIKV from 2018 to 2021 is described below.

Africa

As the continent of origin for Chikungunya, the disease in endemic in Africa with a large number of outbreaks. Between 2017 and 2018, an outbreak occurred in Kenya with 453 infections reported in the capital Mombasa (World Health Organization 2020). From August 2018 onwards, a series of outbreaks were reported in Sudan, Republic of the Congo and Democratic Republic of Congo more than 13,000, 11,000 and 1,000 suspected cases, respectively (Fritz et al. 2019; World Health Organization Africa 2019). Another outbreak was also reported in 2019 in Ethiopia, where more than 50,000 suspected cases were reported (World Health Organization Africa 2019). In Republic of the Congo, a total of 6,149 cases were also reported (Africa Centres for Disease Control and Prevention 2019).

Till 2020, there are about 33 countries that have been affected by CHIKV in Africa (Centre for Disease Control and Prevention 2020a). In the same year, 27,540 Chikungunya cases were reported in Chad, where the first individual who tested positive for CHIKV was a resident from the district of Abeche (Outbreak News Today 2020). However, when investigated, there was no evidence of an imported case scenario (Outbreak News Today 2020). A series of public health responses were summoned to curb further transmission of the virus in Chad (Relief Web 2020). In 2021, there are no updates of cases in Republic of the Congo, Democratic Republic of Congo, Chad, Kenya and Sudan, and there is no data to compare with the previous year (European Centre for Disease Prevention and Control 2021).

Southeast Asia

Malaysia and Thailand were the only countries that record a high number of cases in Southeast Asia (European Centre for Disease Prevention and Control 2021). A total of 990 CHIKV cases were recorded in Malaysia up to December 28, 2019, while 2,556 cases were recorded up to the 51st epidemiological week of 2020 (Ministry of Health 2020; The Star Online

2020). Current data up to April 2021 showed that Malaysia had recorded 388 new cases in Perak and Kuala Lumpur (European Centre for Disease Prevention and Control 2021). From February 16 to March 5, 2021, a total of 56 CHIKV cases were detected in Sentul, Kuala Lumpur, while two others were reported in Lembah Pantai and Titiwangsa (The Star Online 2021). Kuala Lumpur and Putrajaya Health Department director, Datuk Dr Param Jeeth Singh, attributed the outbreak to abandoned houses and clogged drains, which were breeding grounds for *Aedes* mosquitoes. He also said although Chikungunya usually occurred in rural areas, the disease might be transmitted to urban areas due to high morbidity of humans (The Star Online 2021). Two types of virus genotypes had been identified in Malaysia; one being the ECSA genotype, and the other was the Asian genotype isolated from blood samples between 1998 and 2006 (Apandi et al. 2010).

On the other hand, Thailand had recorded 212 cases only in 30 out of the country's 76 provinces in 2020 (European Centre for Disease Prevention and Control 2021). However, there was a huge outbreak of around 15,000 cases in the country, which peaked from June 2018 to January 2019 (Khongwichit et al. 2021). Initially, the outbreak of the virus was reported Satun and Narathiwat (Khongwichit et al. 2021). By December 2018, cases had risen up to 1,759 and the situation became worse from January 2019 onwards. More than 13,000 people were infected in the capital Bangkok (which is a special administrative area apart from the kingdom's 76 provinces) and 60 other provinces (Bureau of Epidemiology 2021; Khongwichit et al. 2021). In fact, most of the cases in 2019 were reported in Bangkok (Khongwichit et al. 2021). The overall morbidity rate of the Thai outbreak was reported to be at 5.40% in 2018 and 19.73% in 2019 (Khongwichit et al. 2021). The phylogenetic analysis of CHIKV in the outbreak revealed a genotype similar to the ECSA strain detected in earlier outbreaks in India from 2008 to 2009, and 2013 (Khongwichit et al. 2021). Hence the 2018/2019 outbreak virus in Thailand could be considered imported from other countries in South Asia and was not prevalent in Thailand (Khongwichit et al. 2021).

South Asia

Being an endemic country, India itself reported for a high number of Chikungunya cases, with current 2021 data showing 1,116 confirmed cases up to April (National Vector Borne Disease Control Programme 2021). The state of Rajasthan recorded the highest number of cases, followed by Karnataka and Maharashtra (National Vector Borne Disease Control Programme 2021). In the previous years, India also reported a total of 6,263 in 2020, 12,205 in 2019 and 9,756 in 2018 (National Vector Borne Disease Control Programme 2021). While cases remained low after 2010, there was a massive outbreak in 2016, with more than 64,000 people falling sick (Hindustan Times 2017). All the outbreaks that took place in 2018 were said to be caused by the Indian Ocean lineage of the ECSA genotype (Newase et al. 2020). Researchers proposed that CHIKV infections after 2005 were probably due to the high susceptibility of Indian citizens compared to foreigners in the region, such as island nations in the Indian Ocean, as they were believed to have achieved herd immunity (Staples et al. 2009; Kumar et al. 2021). It was also concluded that the eastern and the north-eastern Indian states were exposed to higher prevalence of CHIKV infection (Dutta and Mahanta 2006). This was evident in recent years, where neighbouring states like West Bengal, Assam, Tripura and Meghalaya reported their first ever CHIKV infection in 2017 (Hossain et al. 2018).

The Americas

CHIKV cases raised abruptly in the north-eastern region of Brazil in 2019 (da Saude 2020). Phylogenetic analysis of the virus showed that it was the ECSA lineage that could spread rapidly with a high rate of mortality (Xavier et al. 2021). Up to April 2021, Brazil reported 15,708 cases, putting it as a country with the highest number of Chikungunya cases in the world (European Centre for Disease Prevention and Control 2021). This was followed by Bolivia, Colombia, Costa Rica, El Salvador, Paraguay and Venezuela with two-digit cases (European Centre for Disease Prevention and Control 2021). Mexico and Nicaragua reported about two confirmed cases and five suspected cases, respectively (European Centre for Disease Prevention and Control 2021). From 2018 to 2019, CHIKV outbreaks based on CHIKV-DENV coinfections were also observed among children in Cali, Colombia (Castellanos et al. 2021). To help curb Chikungunya in America, an awareness campaign (The Mosquito Action Week) was launched by the Pan American Health Organization to increase the people's knowledge on CHIKV and *Aedes* mosquitoes in the continent (Pan American Health Organization 2020).

CHIKV Burden in Affected Countries and Prevention to Reduce the Burden

Due to the prevalent spread of Chikungunya, this disease has become a burden to many countries and caused severe suffering to people all over the world. At an individual level, acute manifestations such as rashes, arthralgia, fatigue, fever and myalgia are enough to bring extreme pain to patients and reduce their quality of life (Gerardin et al. 2008). In some cases, patients also suffer long-term cerebral disorders that disrupt their mental health and even caused alter their behaviour in some cases (Sanyaolu et al. 2016). With the possibility of causing irreversible long-term effects, Chikungunya should be viewed as a serious threat to humanity as the disease may also affect their social and economic aspects of life. In addition, approximately 75% of patients have reported prolonged or delayed on-set symptoms leading to conditions such as rheumatism (Gerardin et al. 2011; Puntasecca et al. 2021). According to Puntasecca et al. 2021, globally, an average of more than 106,000 disability adjusted life years (DALYS) have lost between 2009 and 2019 because of Chikungunya. A significantly higher DALY rate was observed in the Americas, indicating that the disease is gaining a rapid foothold in the continent (Puntasecca et al. 2021). Following the DALY calculations, the same study proposed for policymakers to take the burden caused by Chikungunya into consideration and alleviate the victims' suffering when discussing policies and measures to contain the disease (Puntasecca et al. 2021).

Chikungunya outbreaks have also driven up public health costs as governments are forced to allocate more resources to combat the disease (UWI Today 2015). Most expenditures will be needed for public education and awareness programmes, besides inspections and vector control activities, such as fogging and spraying (Sanyaolu et al. 2016). In India, after all the outbreaks it suffered, the financial loss faced by the country came to about US$6 million, which are all spent to educate the public on CHIKV (Pan American Health Organization 2006; Krishnamoorthy et al. 2009). A huge loss in national earnings is also observed due to decreased tourism during an outbreak, especially in the Caribbean countries, where governments are forced to provide aid to the people and repair the damage caused by Chikungunya (Krishnamoorthy et al. 2009). For individual patients, losses are incurred due to medical treatment and long-term rehabilitation costs, lost wages and reduced productivity (Sanyaolu et al. 2016). Such hardship may be avoided if not for the prevalence of Chikungunya around the world. This indirectly affects the economic balance of the countries as well.

As vaccines and treatment for the virus are still not available, prevention is the only way to manage the disease. Vector control is one of the best ways to start with, but policymakers have found this method to be very challenging (Volk et al. 2010). Chemical control measures have been employed against *Aedes* mosquitoes, such as environmental sanitation, use of larvicides, repellents and space spraying. (Centre for Disease Control and Prevention 2015). Biological control measures include the use of Wolbachia bacteria to reduce the insects' fertility. Physical controls like lethal ovitraps (originally built to monitor *Aedes* populations) are laced with insecticides and larvicides to attract and destroy female mosquitoes and their eggs (Centre for Disease Control and Prevention 2015; Karthi and Shivakumar 2015). In fact, new approaches such as the pesticide nanoemulsions, novel bioactive molecules and genetic manipulation have been studied to control the population of *Aedes* (Karthi and Shivakumar 2015). A study also suggested the combination of massive spraying and clearing of vector breeding sites to contain Chikungunya from expanding further (Dumont and Chiroleu 2010).

Apart of that, the public needs to be educated on ways to keep safe from mosquito bites and CHIKV transmission. Most of the time, infected individuals are not aware about the symptoms of Chikungunya as compared to dengue. A study in the USA-governed Virgin Islands in the Caribbean, where the disease struck in 2014, reported that only fewer than half of the residents knew about the existence of Chikungunya (Cherry et al. 2016). For an inclusive prevention, community members should play their part in curbing the disease for themselves. In this case, the community needs to be informed and educated on prevention methods. These include wearing covered and light-coloured clothing when going out, using mosquito repellents, utilizing mosquito coils inside the house and using mesh screens for doors and windows to prevent *Aedes* bites (Ministry of Health and Wellness 2021). Community members must also ensure that potential breeding areas, such as flowerpots, old tyres, buckets and rubbish containers inside and outside the house are free of stagnant water (Centre for Disease Control and Prevention 2020b). Health authorities should ensure constant education, communication and dissemination of information regarding the prevention of Chikungunya. Both print and visual media may be well utilised (World Health Organization 2009). Proper control of mosquito population and adequate prevention will make a lot of difference in reducing the spread of the virus.

CONCLUSION

Chikungunya can be classified as among a group of neglected re-emerging diseases that are still prevalent around the world that is endemic in, Africa, America and Asia. Its epidemiology in most continents suggest that the presence of vectors (*Aedes* mosquitoes) and human mobility play an important role in the disease transmission worldwide. Since the nature of the disease is extremely unpredictable, the development of a vaccine or drug becomes a challenge for the scientific community. In this case, improved vector control and prevention measures are the only practical options to stop the spread of the disease. Proper surveillance, awareness campaigns and public cooperation is necessary to keep Chikungunya at bay.

References

Africa Centres for Disease Control and Prevention. (2019). *Chikungunya.* Accessed April 25. https://africacdc.org/disease/chikungunya/.

Apandi, Y., Lau, S. K., Izmawati, N., Amal, N. M., Faudzi, Y., Wan Mansor, Hani, M. H. and Zainah, S. (2010). Identification of chikungunya virus strains circulating in Kelantan, Malaysia in 2009. *Southeast Asian Journal of Tropical Medicine and Public Health*, 41, 1374-1380.

Arankalle, V. A., Shrivastava, S., Cherian, S., Gunjikar, R. S., Walimbe, A. M., Jadhav, S. M., Sudeep, A. B. and Mishra, A. C. (2007). Genetic divergence of Chikungunya viruses in India (1963–2006) with special reference to the 2005–2006 explosive epidemic. *Journal of General Virology*, *88*, 1967-1976.

Aubry, M., Teissier, A., Roche, C., Richard, V., Yan, A. S., Zisou, K., Rouault, E., Maria, V., Lastère, S., Cao-Lormeau, V. M. and Musso, D. (2015). Chikungunya outbreak, French Polynesia, 2014. *Emerging Infectious Diseases*, 21, 724-726.

Bonthius, D. J. (2012). Introduction. *Seminars in Pediatric Neurology*, 19, 87-88.

Bortel, V. W., Dorleans, F., Rosine, J., Blateau, A., Rousset, D., Matheus, S., Leparc-Goffart, I., Flusin, O., Prat, C., Cesaire, R., Najioullah, F., Ardillon, V., Balleydier, E., Carvalho, L., Lemaître, A., Noel, H., Servas, V., Six, C., Zurbaran, M., Leon, L., Guinard, A., van den Kerkhof, J., Henry, M., Fanoy, E., Braks, M., Reimerink, J., Swaan, C., Georges, R., Brooks, L., Freedman, J., Sudre, B. and Zeller, H. (2014). Chikungunya outbreak in the Caribbean region, December 2013 to March 2014, and the significance for Europe. *Eurosurveillance*, 19, 20759.

Bureau of Epidemiology. (2021). *Annual incidence report of Chikungunya virus in Thailand*. Accessed April 25. http://www.boe.moph.go.th/boedb/surdata/disease.php?dcontent=situation&ds=84.

Caglioti, C., Lalle, E., Castilletti, C., Carletti, F., Capobianchi, M. R. and Bordi, L. (2013). Chikungunya virus infection: an overview. *New Microbiologica*, 36, 211-227.

Castellanos, J. E., Jaimes N., Coronel-Ruiza, C., Rojas, J. P., Mejia, L. F., Villarreal, V. H., Maya, L. E., Claros, L. M., Orjuela, C., Calvo, E., Munoz, M. V. and Velandia-Romero, M. L. (2021). Dengue-chikungunya coinfection outbreak in children from Cali, Colombia, in 2018–2019. *International Journal of Infectious Diseases*, 102, 97-102.

Centre for Disease Control and Prevention. (2015). *Chikungunya: vector surveillance and control in the United States*. Accessed May 22. https://www.cdc.gov/chikungunya/pdfs/FINAL-CHIKV-Vector-Surveillance-Control-US05152015.pdf.

Centre for Disease Control and Prevention. (2020a). *Geographic Distribution*. Accessed April 25. https://www.cdc.gov/chikungunya/geo/index.html.

Centre for Disease Control and Prevention. (2020b). *Prevention*. Accessed May 22. https://www.cdc.gov/chikungunya/prevention/ index.html.

Chastel, C. (1963). Human infections in Cambodia by the chikungunya virus or an apparently closely related agent. I. Clinical aspects. Isolations and identification of the viruses. *Bulletin de la Société de Pathologie Exotique*, 56, 892-915. [*Bulletin of the Society of Exotic Pathology*]

Cherry, C. C., Beer, K. D., Fulton, C., Wong, D., Buttke, D., Staples, J. E. and Ellis, E. M. (2016). Knowledge and use of prevention measures for chikungunya virus among visitors - Virgin Islands National Park, 2015. *Travel Medicine and Infectious Disease*, 14, 475–480.

Collao, X., Negredo, A. I., Cano, J., Tenorio, A., de Ory, F., Benito, A., Masia, M. and Sánchez-Seco, M. P. (2010). Different lineages of Chikungunya virus in Equatorial Guinea in 2002 and 2006. *The American Journal of Tropical Medicine and Hygiene*, 82, 505-507.

Crawford, J. E., Alves, J. M., Palmer, W. J., Day, J. P., Sylla, M., Ramasamy, R., Surendran, S. N., Black WC 4th, Pain, A. and Jiggins, F. M. (2017).

Population genomics reveals that an anthropophilic population of Aedes aegypti mosquitoes in West Africa recently gave rise to American and Asian populations of this major disease vector. *BMC Biology*, 15, 16.

da Saúde, M. (2020). Monitoramento dos casos de arboviroses urbanas transmitidas pelo Aedes (Dengue, Chikungunya e Zika), Semanas Epidemiológicas 01 a 52/2019. *Boletim Epidemiológico*, 51, 1-16.

de Lamballerie, X., Leroy, E., Charrel, R. N., Ttsetsarkin K., Higgs, S. and Gould, E. A. (2008). Chikungunya virus adapts to tiger mosquito *via* evolutionary convergence: a sign of things to come? *Virology Journal,* 5, 33.

D'Ortenzio, E., Grandadam, M., Balleydier, E., Jaffar-Bandjee, M. C., Michault, A., Brottet, E., Baville, M. & Filleul, L. (2011). A226V strains of Chikungunya virus, Réunion Island, 2010. *Emerging Infectious Diseases*, 17, 309–311.

Deller, J. J. and Russell, P. K. (1967). An analysis of fevers of unknown origin in American soldiers in Vietnam. *Annals of Internal Medicine*, 66, 1129-1143.

Desdouits, M., Kamgang, B., Berthet, N., Tricou, V., Ngoagouni, C., Gessain, A., Manuguerra, J. C., Nakouné, E. and Kazanji, M. (2015). Genetic characterization of Chikungunya virus in the Central African Republic. *Infection, Genetics and Evolution*, 33, 25-31.

Diallo, M., Thonnon, J., Traore-Lamizana, M. and Fontenille, D. (1999). Vectors of Chikungunya virus in Senegal: Current Data and Transmission Cycles. *The American Society of Tropical Medicine and Hygiene*, 60, 281-286.

Diop, D., Meseznikov, G. and Sanicas, M. (2015). Chikungunya outbreaks from 2000 to 2015: a review. *MOJ Public Health*, 2, 181–187.

Dumont, Y. and Chiroleu, F. (2010). Vector control for the Chikungunya disease. *Mathematical Biosciences and Engineering*, 7, 313-345.

Dutta, P. and Mahanta, J. (2006). Potential vectors of dengue and the profile of dengue in the North- Eastern region of India: An epidemiological perspective. *WHO Regional Office for South-East Asia*, 30, 234-242.

European Centres for Disease Control and Prevention. (2017). *Clusters of autochthonous chikungunya cases in Italy*. Accessed May 26. https://

www.ecdc.europa.eu/sites/portal/files/documents/RRA-chikungunya-Italy-update-9-Oct-2017.pdf.

European Centres for Disease Control and Prevention. (2021). *Chikungunya worldwide overview*. Accessed May 27. https://www. ecdc.europa.eu/en/chikungunya-monthly.

Figueiredo, L. T. M. (2019). Human urban arboviruses can infect wild animals and jump to sylvatic maintenance cycles in South America. *Frontiers in Cellular and Infection Microbiology*, 9, 259.

Fritz, M., Taty Taty, R., Portella, C., Mankou, M., Leroy, E. M. and Becquart, P. (2019). Re-emergence of Chikungunya in the Republic of the Congo in 2019 associated with a possible vector-host switch. *International Journal of Infectious Diseases*, 84, 99-101.

Galan-Huerta, K. A., Rivas-Estilla, A. M., Fernandez-Salas, I., Farfan-Ale, J. A. and Ramos-Jimenez, J. (2015). Chikungunya virus: a general overview. *Medicina Universitaria*, 17, 175-183.

Gérardin, P., Guernier, V., Perrau, J., Fianu, A., Le Roux, K., Grivard, P., Michault, A., de Lamballerie, X., Flahault, A. and Favier, F. (2008). Estimating Chikungunya prevalence in La Réunion Island outbreak by serosurveys: two methods for two critical times of the epidemic. *BMC Infectious Diseases*, 8, 99.

Gérardin, P., Fianu, A., Malvy, D., Mussard, C., Boussaïd, K., Rollot, O., Michault, A., Gaüzere, B. A., Bréart, G. and Favier, F. (2011). Perceived morbidity and community burden after a Chikungunya outbreak: the TELECHIK survey, a population-based cohort study. *BMC Medicine*, 9, 5.

Glushakova, L. G., Alto, B. W., Kim, M. S., Bradley, A., Yaren, O. and Benner, S. A. (2017). Detection of chikungunya viral RNA in mosquito bodies on cationic (Q) paper based on innovations in synthetic biology. *Journal of Virological Methods*, 246, 104-111.

Gobbi, F., Buonfrate, D., Angheben, A., Degani, M. and Bisoffi, C. (2015). Emergence and Surveillance of Chikungunya. *Current Tropical Medicine Reports*, 2, 4-12.

Grandadam, M., Caro, V., Plumet, S., Thiberge, J. M., Souarès, Y, Failloux, A. B., Tolou, H. J., Budelot, M., Cosserat, D., Leparc-Goffart, I. and

Desprès, P. (2011). Chikungunya virus, southeastern France. *Emerging Infectious Diseases*, 17, 910-913.

Griffin, D. E. (2013). 'Alphaviruses.' In: *Fields Virology*, edited by Knipe, D. M, Howley, P. M., Lippincott, Williams and Wilkins.

Gudo, E. S., Black, J. F. P and Cliff, J. L. (2016). Chikungunya in Mozambique: a forgotten history. *PLoS Neglected Tropical Diseases, 10,* e0005001.

Harapan, H., Michie, A., Mudatsir, M., Nusa, R., Yohan, B., Wagner, A. L., Sasmono, R. T. and Imrie, A. (2019). Chikungunya virus infection in Indonesia: a systematic review and evolutionary analysis. *BMC Infectious Diseases,* 19, 243.

Hindustan Times. (2017). *Chikungunya Virus Emerges as Bigger Threat to People in North India*. Accessed May 27. https://www.hindustantimes.com/health/caution-chikungunya-virus-emerges-as-bigger-threat-to-people-in-north-india/story-YDjbT4Oae3xSESx8UZ6yhO.html.

Hossain, M. S., Hasan, M. M., Islam, M. S., Islam, S., Mozaffor, M., Khan, M. A. S., Ahmed, N., Akhtar, W., Chowdhury, S., Arafat, S. M. Y., Khaleque, M. A., Khan, Z. J., Dipta, T. F., Asna, S. M. Z. H., Hossain, M. A., Aziz, K. S., Mosabbir, A. A. and Raheem, E. (2018). Chikungunya outbreak (2017) in Bangladesh: Clinical profile, economic impact and quality of life during the acute phase of the disease. *PLoS Neglected Tropical Diseases*, 12, e0006561.

James, S. L., Abate, D., Abate, K. H., Abay, S. M., Abbafati, C., Abbasi, N., Abbastabar, H., Abd-Allah, F., Abdela, J., Abdelalim, A. and Abdollahpour, I. (2018). Global, regional, and national incidence, prevalence, and years lived with disability for 354 diseases and injuries for 195 countries and territories, 1990–2017: a systematic analysis for the Global Burden of Disease Study 2017. *The Lancet*, 392, 1789-1858.

Johnson, B. W., Russell, B. J. and Goodman, C. H. (2016). Laboratory Diagnosis of Chikungunya Virus Infections and Commercial Sources for Diagnostic Assays. *The Journal of Infectious Diseases*, 214, S471-S474.

Jupp, P. and McIntosh, B. (1988). 'Chikungunya virus disease.' In *The arboviruses: epidemiology and ecology*, edited by Monath T., Boca Rotan Florida: CRC Press, 137-157.

Karthi S. and Shivakumar M. S. (2015). Vector control in chikungunya and other arboviruses. In: *Current topics in chikungunya*, edited by Rodriguez-Morales, A. J., IntechOpen, 123–32.

Khongwichit, S., Chansaenroj, J., Thongmee, T., Benjamanukul, S., Wanlapakorn, N., Chirathaworn, C. and Poovorawan, Y. (2021). Large-scale outbreak of Chikungunya virus infection in Thailand, 2018–2019. *PloS ONE*, 16, e0247314.

Kosasih, H., de Mast, Q., Widjaja, S., Sudjana, P., Antonjaya, U., Ma'roef, C., Riswari, S. F., Porter, K. R., Burgess, T. H., Alisjahbana, B. and van der Ven, A. (2013). Evidence for endemic chikungunya virus infections in Bandung, Indonesia. *PLoS Neglected Tropical Diseases*, *7*, e2483.

Krishnamoorthy, K., Harichandrakumar, K. T., Krishna Kumari, A. and Das, L. K. (2009). Burden of chikungunya in India: estimates of disability adjusted life years (DALY) lost in 2006 epidemic. *Journal of Vector Borne Diseases*, 46, 26-35.

Kumar, M. S., Kamaraj, P., Khan, S. A., Allam, R. R., Barde, P. V., Dwibedi, B., Kanungo, S., Mohan, U., Mohanty, S. S., Roy, S., Sagar, V., Savargaonkar, D., Tandale, B. V., Topno, R. K., Kumar, C. P. G., Sabarinathan, R., Kumar, V. S., Bitragunta, S., Grover, G. S., Lakshmi, P. V. M., Mishra, C. M., Sadhukhan, P., Sahoo, P. K., Singh, S. K., Yadav, C. P., Dinesh, E. R., Karunakaran, T., Govindhasamy, G., Rajasekar, T. D., Jeyakumar, A., Suresh, A., Augustine, D., Kumar, P. A., Kumar, R., Dutta, S., Toteja, G. S., Gupta, N., Clapham, H. E., Mehendale, S. M. and Murhekar, M. V. (2021). Seroprevalence of chikungunya virus infection in India, 2017: a cross-sectional population-based serosurvey. *Lancet Microbe*, 2, 41-47.

Laras, K., Sukri, N. C., Larasati, R. P., Bangs, M. J., Kosim, R., Wandra, T., Master, J., Kosasih, H., Hartati, S., Beckett, C. and Sedyaningsih, E. R. (2005). Tracking the re-emergence of epidemic chikungunya virus in Indonesia. *Transactions of the Royal Society of Tropical Medicine and Hygiene*, 99, 128-141.

Leparc-Goffart, I., Nougairede, A., Cassadou, S., Prat, C. and de Lamballerie, X. (2014). Chikungunya in the Americas. *The Lancet*, 383, 514.

Mason, P. J. and Haddow A. J. (1957). An epidemic of virus disease in Southern Province, Tanganyika Territory, in 1952-53; an additional note on Chikungunya virus isolations and serum antibodies. *Transactions of the Royal Society of Tropical Medicine and Hygiene*, 51, 238-240.

Matusali, G., Colavita, F., Bordi, L., Lalle, E., Ippolito, G., Capobianchi, M. R. and Castilletti, C. (2019). Tropism of the Chikungunya Virus. *Viruses*, 11, 175.

Mendis, N. M. P. (1967). Epidemiology of dengue-like fever in Ceylon. *Ceylon Medical Journal*, 12, 67-74.

Ministry of Health. (2020). '*Situasi demasa demam denggi, zika dan chikungunya di Malaysia*.' Accessed May 19. http://www.myhealth.gov.my/wp-content/uploads/PS_KPK_Denggi-Zika-Di-Malaysia-ME-51.2020.pdf.

Ministry of Health and Wellness. (2021). *Chikungunya awareness and prevention*. Accessed May 22. https://www.moh.gov.jm/edu-resources/chikungunya-awareness-prevention/.

Mohamat, S. A., Mat N. F. C., Barkadle, N. I., Jusoh, T. N. A. M. and Shueb, R. H. (2020). Chikungunya and alternative treatment from natural products: a review. *Malaysian Journal of Medicine and Health Sciences*, 16, 3014-3111.

Mombouli, J. V., Bitsindou, P., Elion, D. O., Grolla, A., Feldmann, H., Niama, F. R., Parra, H. J. and Munster, V. J. (2013). Chikungunya virus infection, Brazzaville, Republic of Congo, 2011. *Emerging Infectious Diseases*, *19*, 1542.

National Vector Borne Disease Control Programme. (2021). *Epidemiological profile of chikungunya fever in the country since 2015*. Accessed May 21. https://nvbdcp.gov.in/index4.php?lang=1&level=0&linkid=486&lid=3765.

Newase, P., More, A., Patil, J., Patil, P., Jadhav, S., Alagarasu, K., Shah, P., Parashar, D. and Cherian, S. S. (2020). Chikungunya phylogeography reveals persistent global transmissions of the Indian Ocean Lineage from India in association with mutational fitness. *Infection, Genetics and Evolution*, 82, 104289.

Outbreak News Today. (2020). *Chikungunya outbreak: 27,540 cases reported in Chad, Most in Abeche*. Accessed May 21. http://outbreaknewstoday.com/chikungunya-outbreak-27540-cases-reported-in-chad-most-in-abeche-78170/.

Pan American Health Organization. (2006). *Report of the Caribbean Commission on health and development*. Accessed May 19. https://www.who.int/macrohealth/action/PAHO_Report.pdf.

Pan American Health Organization. (2014a). *Number of reported cases of chikungunya fever in the Americas – EW 26 (June 27, 2014)*. Accessed May 25. https://www.paho.org/hq/dmdocuments/2014/2014-jun-27-cha-CHIKV-authoch-imported-cases-ew-26.pdf.

Pan American Health Organization. (2014b). *Number of reported cases of chikungunya fever in the Americas – EW 30 (July 25, 2014)*. Accessed May 25. https://www.paho.org/hq/dmdocuments/2014/2014-jul-25-cha-CHIKV-authoch-imported-cases-ew-30.pdf.

Pan American Health Organization. (2014c). *Number of reported cases of chikungunya fever in the Americas – EW 47 (November 21, 2014)*. Accessed May 25. https://www.paho.org/hq/dmdocuments/2014/2014-nov-21-cha-chikungunya-cases-ew-47.pdf.

Pan American Health Organization. (2020). *Caribbean Mosquito Awareness Week 2020*. Accessed April 21. https://www.paho.org/en/campaigns/caribbean-mosquito-awareness-week-2020.

Parreira, R., Centeno-Lima, S., Lopes, A., Portugal-Calisto, D., Constantino, A. and Nina, J. (2014). Dengue virus serotype 4 and chikungunya virus coinfection in a traveller returning from Luanda, Angola, January 2014. *Eurosurveillance*, *19*, 20730.

Paupy, C., Kassa Kassa, F., Caron, M., Nkoghé, D. and Leroy, E. M. (2012). A chikungunya outbreak associated with the vector *Aedes albopictus* in remote villages of Gabon. *Vector-borne and Zoonotic Diseases*, 12, 167-169.

Pialoux, G., Gauzere, B. B., Jaureguiberry, S. and Strobel, M. (2007). Chikungunya, an epidemic arbovirosis. *The Lancet Infectious Diseases*, 7, 319-327.

Powers, A. M. and Logue, C. H. (2007). Changing patterns of chikungunya virus: re-emergence of a zoonotic arbovirus. *Journal of General Virology*, 88, 2363-2377.

Puntasecca, C. J., King, C. H. and LaBeaud, A. D. (2021). Measuring the global burden of chikungunya and Zika viruses: a systematic review. *PLoS Neglected Tropical Diseases.* 15, e0009055.

Qiaoli, Z., Jianfeng, H., De, W., Zijun, W., Xinguang, Z., Haojie, Z., Fan, D., Zhiquan, L., Shiwen, W., Zhenyu, H. and Yonghui, Z. (2012). Maiden outbreak of chikungunya in Dongguan city, Guangdong province, China: epidemiological characteristics. *PloS ONE*, *7*, e42830.

Reiter P, Sprenger D. (1987). The used tire trade: a mechanism for the worldwide dispersal of container breeding mosquitoes. *Journal of the American Mosquito Control Association*, 3, 494-501.

Renault, P., Solet, J. L., Sissoko, D., Balleydier, E., Larrieu, S., Filleul, L., Lassalle, C., Thiria, J., Rachou, E., de Valk, H., Ilef, D., Ledrans, M., Quatresous, I., Quenel, P. and Pierre, V. (2007). A major epidemic of chikungunya virus infection on Reunion Island, France, 2005-2006. *The American Journal of Tropical Medicine and Hygiene*, 77, 727-731.

Relief Web. (2020). *Chikungunya – Chad: Disease outbreak news, 24 September 2020*. Accessed April 25. https://reliefweb.int/report/chad/chikungunya-chad-disease-outbreak-news-24-september-2020.

Rezza, G., Nicoletti, L., Angelini, R., Romi, R., Finarelli, A. C., Panning, M., Cordioli, P., Fortuna, C., Boros, S., Magurano, F. and Silvi, G. (2007). Infection with chikungunya virus in Italy: an outbreak in a temperate region. *The Lancet*, 370, 1840-1846.

Sam, I. C., Loong, S. K., Michael, J. C., Chua, C. L., Sulaiman, W. Y. W., Vythilingam, I., Chan, S. Y., Chiam, C. W., Yeong, Y. S., AbuBakar, S. and Chan, Y. F. (2012). Genotypic and phenotypic characterization of Chikungunya virus of different genotypes from Malaysia. *PloS one*, 7, e50476.

Sanyaolu, A., Okorie, C., Badaru, O., Wynveen, E., White, S., Wallace, W., Aki, J., Freeze, A., Kamel, A., Madonna, M., Mathur, A., Moran, R. and Perry, C. (2016). Chikungunya epidemiology: a global perspective. *SM Journal of Public Health and Epidemiology*, 2, 1028.

Saswat, T., Kumar, A., Kumar, S., Mamidi, P., Muduli, S., Debata, N. K., Pal, N. S., Pratheek, B. M., Chattopadhyay, S. and Chattopadhyay, S. (2015). High rates of co-infection of Dengue and Chikungunya virus in Odisha and Maharashtra, India during 2013. *Infection, Genetics and Evolution*, 35, 134-141.

Staples, J. E., Breiman, R. F. and Powers, A. M. (2009). Chikungunya fever: An epidemiological review of a re-emerging infectious disease. *Clinical Infectious Diseases*, 49, 942-948.

Staples, J. E., Hills, S. L. and Powers, A. M. (2020). Chikungunya. In: *CDC Yellow Book 2020*, Oxford University Press.

Sergon, K., Njuguna, C., Kalani, R., Ofula, V., Onyango, C., Konongoi, L. S., Bedno, S., Burke, H., Dumilla, A. M., Konde, J., Njenga, M. K., Sang, R. and Breiman, R. F. (2004). Seroprevalence of Chikungunya virus (CHIKV) infection on Lamu Island, Kenya. *American Journal of Tropical Medicine and Hygiene*, 78, 333-337.

Shiferaw, B., Lam, P., Tuthill, S., Choudhry, H., Syed, S., Ahmed, S. and Yasmin, T. (2015). The chikungunya epidemic: a look at five cases. *IDCases*, *2*, 89–91.

Simon, F., Javelle, E., Oliver, M., Leparc-Goffart, I. and Marimoutou, C. (2011). Chikungunya virus infection. *Current Infectious Disease Reports*, 13, 218-228.

Sowards, W. (2019). *Where did chikungunya come from*?. Accessed April 25. https://www.passporthealthusa.com/2019/04/where-did-chikungunya-come-from/.

Thaung, U., Ming, C. K., Swe, T. and Thein, S. (1975). Epidemiological features of dengue and chikungunya infections in Burma. *The Southeast Asian Journal of Tropical Medicine and Public Health*, 6, 276-283.

The Star Online. (2020). *Dengue cases hit beyond 130,000 cases last year*. Accessed May 27. https://www.thestar.com.my/news/nation/2020/01/03/dengue-cases-hit-beyond-130000-cases-last-year.

The Star Online. (2021). *On alert following chikungunya outbreak.* Accessed May 20. https://www.thestar.com.my/metro/metro-news/2021/03/09/on-alert-following-chikungunya-outbreak.

UWI Today. (2015). *The chikungunya effect.* Accessed May 18. https://sta.uwi.edu/uwitoday/archive/february_2015/article17.asp.

Valentine, M. J., Murdock, C. C. and Kelly, P. J. (2019). Sylvatic cycles of arboviruses in non-human primates. *Parasites Vectors*, 12, 463.

Vega-Rua, A., Zouache, K., Caro, V., Diancourt, L., Delaunay, P., Grandadam, M. and Failloux, A. B. (2013). High efficiency of temperate *Aedes albopictus* to transmit chikungunya and dengue viruses in the Southeast of France. *PloS ONE*, *8*, e59716.

Vega-Rúa, A., Lourenço-de-Oliveira, R., Mousson, L., Vazeille, M., Fuchs, S., Yébakima, A., Gustave, J., Girod, R., Dusfour, I., Leparc-Goffart, I., Vanlandingham, D. L., Huang, Y. J., Lounibos, L. P., Mohamed Ali, S., Nougairede, A., de Lamballerie, X. and Failloux, A. B. (2015). Chikungunya virus transmission potential by local *Aedes* mosquitoes in the Americas and Europe. *PLoS Neglected Tropical Diseases,* 9, e0003780.

Volk, S. M., Chen, R., Tsetsarkin, K. A., Adams, A. P., Garcia, T. I., Sall, A. A., Nasar, F., Schuh, A. J., Holmes, E. C., Higgs, S., Maharaj, P. D., Brault, A. C. and Weaver, S. C. (2010). Genome-scale phylogenetic analyses of chikungunya virus reveal independent emergences of recent epidemics and various evolutionary rates. *Journal of Virology*, 84, 6497-6504.

Wahid, B., Ali, A. and Idrees, M. (2017). Global expansion of chikungunya virus: mapping the 64-year history. *International Journal of Infectious Diseases*, 58, 69-76.

Weaver, S. C., Osorio, J. E., Livengood, J. A., Chen, R. and Stinchcomb, D. T. (2012). Chikungunya virus and prospects for a vaccine. *Expert Review of Vaccines*, 11, 1087-1101.

Weinbren, M. P., Haddow, A. J. and Williams, M. C. (1958). *Transactions of the Royal Society of Tropical Medicine and Hygiene*, 52, 253-258.

World Health Organization. (2006). Outbreak news: chikungunya and dengue, south-west Indian Ocean. *The Weekly Epidemiological Record*, 81, 106-108.

World Health Organization. (2009). *Guidelines for prevention and control of chikungunya fever*. Accessed May 22. file:///C:/Users/Z/Downloads/B4289.pdf.

World Health Organization. (2016). *Chikugunya – Argentina*. Accessed April 20. https://www.who.int/csr/don/14-march-2016-chikungunya-argentina/en/.

World Health Organization Africa. (2019). *Weekly bulletin on outbreaks and other emergencies – week 28, 8–14 July 2019*. Accessed April 18. https://apps.who.int/iris/bitstream/handle/10665/325864/OEW28-0814072019.pdf.

World Health Organization. (2020). *Chikugunya.* Accessed April 18. https://www.who.int/news-room/fact-sheets/detail/chikungunya.

World Health Organization. (2021). *Chikugunya*. Accessed April 20. https://www.who.int/denguecontrol/arbo-viral/other_arboviral_chikungunya/en/.

Xavier, J., Fonseca, V., Bezerra, J. F., Alves, M. M., Mares-Guia, M. A., Claro, I. M., Jesus, R., Adelino, T., Araújo, E., Cavalcante, K. R. L. J., Tosta, S., Souza, T. R., Cruz, F., E., M., Fabri, A. A., Oliveira, E. C., Moura, N. F. O., Said, R. F. C., Albuquerque, C. F. C., Azevedo, V., Oliveira, T., Filippis, A. M. B., Cunha, R. V., Luz, K. G., Giovanetti, M. and Alcantara, L. C. J. (2021). Chikungunya virus ECSA lineage reintroduction in the northeasternmost region of Brazil. *International Journal of Infectious Diseases*, 105, 120-123.

Zeller, H., Bortel, W. V. and Sudre, B. (2016). Chikungunya: its history in Africa and Asia and its spread to new regions in 2013–2014. *The Journal of Infectious Diseases*, 214, 436-440.

In: Chikungunya
Editor: Phillip Galvan
ISBN: 978-1-53619-978-9

Chapter 2

GEOGRAPHICAL DISTRIBUTION, TRANSMISSION AND ALTERNATIVE HOSTS OF CHIKUNGUNYA VIRUS

Caroline Wasonga*, PhD
Department of Biochemistry, University of Nairobi,
Nairobi, Kenya

ABSTRACT

Chikungunya is a re-emerging acute febrile illness whose outbreaks have been documented globally. Chikungunya outbreaks have occurred in several continents and countries with the first Chikungunya virus being isolated from the serum of a febrile patient in Tanzania in 1953. From 1953 several suspected and laboratory confirmed cases have been reported in East Africa, Indian Ocean Islands, Asia, Europe, North America and the Caribbean Islands. During these outbreaks, some fatalities associated with this outbreaks have been documented like in Reunion Island outbreak of 2005. The spread of Chikungunya virus in a number countries occurred due to the arrival of Chikungunya infected travelers from endemic countries, for example, India and Europe received infected travelers from

* Corresponding Author's E-mail: cwasonga@uonbi.ac.ke.

the Indian Ocean Islands. As recent as 2020, Chikungunya outbreaks are still being reported.

The distribution of Chikungunya has been associated with new vectors that can competitively transmit this virus. Chikungunya virus transmission occurs in two cycles: sylvatic and urban cycle. In Africa, the virus is maintained in a sylvatic cycle which includes non-human primates (chimpanzees, monkeys and baboons) and different species of mosquitoes that dwell in the forests. Chikungunya virus may have evolved from these forest-dwelling mosquitoes in Central Africa, and then adapted to an urban cycle as it spread from Africa through the Indian Ocean Islands, then to Asia. In the urban cycle which has been reported in Asia and urban settings, the virus is transmitted via *Aedes aegypti and Aedes albopictus* mosquitoes to human through the bite of an infected mosquito. Transmission and spread of Chikungunya and other viral diseases should be closely monitored by performing routine surveillance to prevent economic losses that may come with disease outbreaks.

Keywords: Chikungunya virus, transmission, reservoir, outbreak, geographical distribution

INTRODUCTION

Alphaviruses belong to the family Togaviridae and are enveloped, single-stranded, positive-sense RNA viruses. Alphaviruses are arboviruses that are maintained in non-human primates, wildlife, rodents and birds outside epidemics. These diseases can spill over to human beings after being bitten by infected mosquitoes, or when alphaviruses emerge to cause epizootics and epidemics. Five types of alphaviruses that commonly infect people in the tropics and are capable of transmitting and disseminating the virus are chikungunya, Venezuelan equine encephalitis, Mayaro, Ross River and O'nyong-nyong viruses.

The name Chikungunya is derived from the Makonde word which means "that which bends up" in reference to the stooped posture developed as a result of the arthritic symptom of the disease. Joint pain, which is characteristic of Chikungunya virus (CHIKV) infection, may lead to difficulty in standing straight or walking and general malaise. Other symptoms of Chikungunya include fever, headache, muscle pain, joint swelling and a rash. These symptoms typically occur two to twelve days after exposure to the virus. Symptoms usually improve within one week, occasionally, the joint pain may last for months or years and can incapacitate a patient, keeping the victims away from their daily household and economic activities.

Being an alphavirus, Chikungunya virus has an RNA genome that is at least 11.8 kilobases, functions as a messenger RNA (mRNA) and begins replication and translation upon entry into a cell. The non-structural proteins (nsP1–nsP4) required for replication are encoded at the 5' end of the genome, and the structural proteins are encoded at the 3' end (Griffin, 2001).

Chikungunya virus is detected by virus isolation, reverse transcription-Polymerase chain reaction (RT-PCR) and by serological assays. During routine cell culture and isolation of viruses, through RT-PCR and sequencing of the identified isolates, virus evolution can be monitored by screening for plaque variants and mutations from isolates from human and mosquitoes. These virus strains could have important implications for disease severity, increased transmission and lead to devastating outbreaks. Other than testing for the CHIKV, CHIKV specific antibodies can also be tested using serological assays to assess circulation of this virus after the vireamic phase, which is short-lived. Serological assays can be done using Enzyme-Linked immunosorbent assay.

Chikungunya is not typically a life threatening disease as most patients fully recover from it. Widespread Chikungunya outbreaks can have serious consequences such as reduced productivity at personal, household and community level, a strain in the healthcare system, a negative impact on the economy of the country, and exacerbation of poverty particularly in individuals from low and middle economic backgrounds. It is important to put in place preventive measures like routine surveillance of the disease by assessing its circulation in human and other hosts, and monitor vector abundance and diversity, and enhance the capacity of the healthcare systems, just in case an outbreak occurs.

Geographical Distribution of Chikungunya

There has been a re-emergence of enormous outbreaks of Chikungunya in the 21st century, which has spread across a number of continents, ranging from Africa, including East Africa and the Indian Ocean Islands, Asia including India, Europe, Australia, North Americas, and the Caribbean Islands.

It has been speculated that Chikungunya infections were reported for the first time around 1779. This initial outbreak occurred in Dutch East Indies, specifically in Batavia, which is located in the present day Jakarta, Indonesia, where the patients presented with Dengue fever-like symptoms. In this outbreak, a Dutch physician reported febrile illness characterized with knuckle or joint pain, acute fever, rash and chronic arthralgia. Outbreaks with similar symptoms occurred in Zanzibar in 1823 and 1870, in India it occurred at different times, that is from 1824 to 1964 and in the south-eastern U.S. in 1827-28 (Carey, 1971). In the following sub-sections, we shall explore the reported episodes of Chikungunya Outbreaks in different continents including Africa, Asia, Europe, and the Americas.

Chikungunya Outbreaks in Africa and Indian Ocean Regions

In 1952, Marion Robinson and Lumsden (Robinson, 1955 and Lumsden, 1955), reported a Chikungunya outbreak in Makonde Plateau, which is located along the Tanganyika and Mozambique border. The following year in 1953 Chikungunya virus was isolated for the first time by Ross during an outbreak in Tanzania, specifically Newala district (Ross, 1956).

After the first virus isolation, subsequent CHIKV isolations were done in many countries between the 1960 all through to 1990. These countries were mainly in Central, Southern and West Africa. In Central Africa, the countries included Kenya, Uganda, Democratic Republic of Congo (DRC) and Sudan. Southern African countries included Malawi, Zimbabwe, and South Africa. Lastly, in West Africa, the countries included were Benin,

Nigeria, Senegal, the Republic of Guinea and Cote d`Ivoire (Powers and Logue, 2007).

An outbreak of Chikungunya in Lamu Island, located in Coastal Kenya, occurred in May 2004 and peaked in July the same year, 1,300 patients were infected with the virus, and this constituted approximately 75% of the total population on the island. Thankfully, no deaths related to the outbreak were reported. Among the symptomatic patients, 84% were absent from work or school due to prolonged illness. In November of the same year, a Chikungunya outbreak was reported in Mombasa, and genetic analysis of the circulating virus shown that the virus strain that circulated in Mombasa was related to the one identified in Lamu. (Kariuki et al., 2008).

The presence of Chikungunya in the Comoros Island was reported in February 2005, peaking in March the same year. A total of 5,202 cases were laboratory confirmed, representing 63% of the population. No deaths associated with this outbreak were reported (Sergon et al., 2008). Due to previous outbreaks of Dengue in 1948, 1984, and 1993, when an outbreak occurred in Comoros in 2015, it was believed that this outbreak was caused by dengue virus. However, after laboratory testing of the patients sera by serology and molecular analysis, it was confirmed that the virus responsible for this outbreak was CHIKV (Sergon et al., 2008). Later in March of 2005, some of the infected patients in Comoros Island travelled to Re union Island, becoming the first documented cases in Reunion Island (Schuffenecker et al., 2006). In March and July 2005 and January 2006, after arrival of affected travelers from Comoros Island, a massive outbreak of CHIKV occurred in Reunion Island, where 244,000 cases were reported and this cases represented 40% of the population. Some of the casualties associated with the Re-Union Island outbreak were the elderly population, where 213 persons were lost (Schuffenecker et al., 2006, Renault et al., 2007). From Reunion Island, genetic evidence showed that the CHIKV spread to Seychelles, Mauritius, Madagascar, Mayotte, and the Maldives (Powers, 2011). Chikungunya outbreaks were also reported in Sudan (2018) and Chad (2020).

Chikungunya Circulation in Kenya during the Inter-Epidemic Period

Circulating immunoglobulin G (IgG) has been reported in coastal and Lake Basin regions of Kenya. Table 1 shows the seroprevalence of Chikungunya in Kenya. It is interesting that Kisumu and Busia are both located on the shores of Lake Victoria.

Seroprevalence data from a few studies have confirmed that Chikungunya occurred in different parts of Kenya and the circulating antibodies could have been detected by ELISA during the inter-epidemic periods. In Busia County in Kenya, a prevalence of 59.9% in 2004 and 11.5% in 2010 was reported (Sutherland et al., 2011, Mwongula et al., 2013). A prevalence of 37% was observed in Coastal Kenya (24.77%) in 2004 (Mease et al., 2011) and in Kisumu county lowlands (42%) in children (Sutherland et al., 2011). This demonstrates that CHIKV is circulating in the population without being detected or reaching epidemic levels.

The circulation of CHIKV specific antibodies indicates that the populations in these regions have had previous exposure to CHIKV and the antibodies generated have persisted in the population from between one week to several months/years. In 2013, when there was a reported Dengue outbreak in Kenya, Chikungunya was found to be circulating during this outbreak with acute cases being reported mainly along the coastal parts of Kenya. From the seroprevalence data, the populations at risk of Chikungunya infection were the elderly and children (Wasonga et al., 2015). Infections were also high among those that are immunocompromised like expecting mothers and individuals with complications arising from other ailment like arthritis.

The reason for the prevalence of the disease in the coast and western parts of Kenya is unclear. Considering that *Aedes* (*Ae.) aegypti* is well distributed throughout Kenya and that the vector distribution does not limit the disease. It is hypothesized that the climatic conditions especially temperature and humidity could be the main factor (Lutomiah et al., 2013). Therefore, Kenya could be at risk of CHIKV outbreaks because of active transmission in endemic regions, movement of people across the country for trading, education and economic opportunities, and great variability in climate, which could result in temperature and humidity conditions that could create favorable conditions for *Aedes* mosquitoes breeding in almost any part of the country.

Table 1. Seroprevalence of Chikungunya in Kenya

Regions	Sites	Year of study	Target population	% Seropre-valence	References
Western Kenya	Busia District	2010	Pyretic children	11.5	Mwongula et al., 2013
	Busia District	2004	Adults	59.9	Mease et al., 2011
	Kisumu District	2004	children	42.0	Sutherland et al., 2011
	Nyanza and Central Kenya	1966-1968	All age-groups	54.6	Geser et al., 1970
Coastal Kenya	Msambweni district	2000-2003	Pregnant women	37.0	Sutherland et al., 2011
	Malindi District	2004	Adults	24.8	Mease et al., 2011
	Coastal Kenya	1987	adults	0.7	Morrill et al., 1991
	Malindi District	1966-1968	All age-groups	50.8	Geser et al., 1970
Rift Valley	Nandi District	2004	children	0.0	Sutherland et al., 2011
Eastern Kenya	Samburu District	2004	Adults	0.0	Mease et al., 2011
	Kitui	1966-1968	All age-groups	1.0	Geser et al., 1970

Chikungunya Outbreak in Asia and Europe

India had its first Chikungunya outbreak in Kolkata in 1963 (Arankalle et al., 2007) followed by outbreaks in other parts of the country. The outbreaks in Chennai, Pondicherry, and Vellore were reported in 1964. In 1965, there were outbreaks in Kakinada, Visakhapatnam, Rajahmundry, and Nagpur, followed by Barsai in 1973 (Arankalle et al., 2007). After 32 years, massive CHIKV infection re-emerged in India between 2005 and 2008. These infections affected 1.3 million patients in 13 different states (Ravi, 2006). In Sri-Lanka, Chikungunya re-emerged in October 2006 and June 2008 with more than 40,000 suspected cases reported after a period of 40 years (Hapuarachchi et al., 2008). In 2006, 7000 cases were reported in Malaysia (AbuBakar et al., 2007). In Singapore a Chikungunya outbreak occurred in January 2008 (Leo et al., 2009). In the Maldives, atleast 12,000 Chikungunya cases were reported between 2006 and 2007 (Yoosuf et al., 2008). In Thailand some cases were reported between 2008 and 2009 (Theamboonlers et al., 2009).

In 2006 and 2007, CHIKV infections were confirmed in travelers returning to Europe including, Belgium, United Kingdom, Germany, Italy, Spain, Switzerland and France among other countries. Over the same period, CHIKV infections were also confirmed in travelers returning to Canada, Corsica, Japan, Australia, Hong Kong, Taiwan, Singapore, Sri-Lanka, Gabon and the USA. These cases were directly associated with the return of symptomatic travelers, who had recently arrived from endemic regions in the Islands of the Indian Ocean and Asia (Lanciotti et al., 2007 and Warner et al., 2006). In 2007, Autochthonous transmission was reported, with at least 254 cases being locally acquired in Northern Italy (Rezza et al., 2007). Autochthonous transmission is where the infection is transmitted locally or in the same place between native individuals and not from migrants.

Chikungunya outbreak was reported in New Guinea in 2012 (Horwood et al., 2013), in China in 2010 (Wu et al., 2013) and in New Caledonia in 2011 (Dupont-Rouzeyrol et al., 2012). Europe had a confirmed Chikungunya case in France in 2014 and in 2017, locally transmitted cases were reported in France and Italy. Between 2018 and 2019, the incidents of Chikungunya were at least 15,000 across 60 different provinces in Thailand (Khongwichit et al., 2021). Between February and March, 2021, 115 cases were reported in Malaysia and 136 cases in Thailand with no associated deaths. These Chikungunya numerous outbreaks have become an issue of public health concern in several countries, due to the increasing number of Chikungunya infections reported globally.

Chikungunya Virus Spread in the Americas

Prior to the CHIKV outbreak in the Caribbean island in 2013, all reported cases in the Caribbean Island were imported from other countries which had previously reported Chikungunya outbreaks outside the Americas and no local transmission of the virus had been reported in areas that were endemic to Dengue. These areas had *Ae. aegpyti* and *Ae. albopictus* mosquitoes inhabiting their environs (Lanciotti et al., 2007). The Indian Ocean lineage of CHIKV that is mainly transmitted by *Ae. albopictus* had been detected in both temperate regions like Italy and Spain (Rezza et al., 2007), and tropical regions like India. However, non-exposure of the Americans to CHIKV, made them susceptible and at risk of a Chikungunya outbreak because of the presence of both *Ae. aegpyti* and *Ae. albopictus* in the region, and a surge in the number of infected travelers arriving into the Caribbean and/or Latin America. (Weaver and Reisen 2009). Indeed in October, 2013, CHIKV circulation was detected in Saint Martin Island with 4,300 confirmed cases (Leparc-Goffart et al., 2014)

Local transmission in French Guiana which is located in the South American mainland, had 176 suspected cases of Chikungunya reported. The CHIKV strain that was detected in these outbreaks in the Americas, was the strain that gets transmitted more efficiently through *Ae. aegpyti* than in *Ae. albopictus* (Tsetsarkin et al., 2007). Since transmission of CHIKV occurred in the Americas through *Ae. aegpyti,* this limited the geographical spread of this virus, particularly in temperate climates where mosquitoes do not normally thrive. Since 1970s, millions of people have been at risk of CHIKV re-infection in most of the tropic and sub tropic regions of Latin America, due to persistence of the virus in Southern part of the United States. (Gubler 2011). The first case of local transmission of the virus in the American continent was reported in 2013, in Saint Martin and Martinique Islands.

Chikungunya cases were reported in several Islands in the Caribbean in January 2014. These Islands included, Guadeloupe, Dominica, the Grenadines Anguilla, Saint Barthelemy, Guadeloupe, and Dominican Republic. Later in 2014, cases were reported in the Pacific islands, which included Kiribati, Cook Islands, American Samoa, Marshall Islands, Samoa and French Polynesia. Within 4 months, more than 30,000 cases were reported in the Caribbean Island and the vector likely responsible for this outbreak was *Ae. aegypti* mosquitoes, since this was the only circulating vector within the Islands at that time (Leparc-Goffart et al., 2014).

Between January and March 2021, in the Americas and the Caribbean, Chikungunya suspected cases were reported in a number of countries including, Bolivia (43 cases and 10 laboratory-confirmed cases), Brazil (8 841 cases, 1793 of which were laboratory-confirmed), Colombia (five cases), Costa Rica (nine cases), El Salvador (14 cases), Guatemala (52 cases), Mexico (one confirmed case), Nicaragua (four cases), Paraguay (49 cases, two laboratory-confirmed) and Venezuela (nine cases). (https://www.ecdc.europa.eu/en/chikungunya-monthly. Accessed on 18th May 2021).

Since CHIKV is transmitted by mosquitoes, local transmission can occur when the vector is introduced to a new area where it can survive or the vector is introduced into an area where it had previously been eliminated. Transmission also occurs when the environmental factors like precipitation, temperature and humidity favor vector survival in an area where the vector could not thrive previously. The re-emergence of these vectors can be pointers to an impending outbreak of CHIKV in an area that has been free from the disease.

Transmission of Chikungunya Virus

Chikungunya is a viral disease transmitted to humans by infected *Aedes* Species of mosquitoes. In the natural habitat, CHIKV exists in two transmission cycles, Sylvatic and urban transmission cycles.

Sylvatic Cycle of Chikungunya Virus in Africa

As a zoonotic virus, CHIKV is mainly maintained in sylvatic cycles with occasional spill over to human leading to local outbreaks. In Africa, CHIKV circulates in a sylvatic cycle and involves viruses that circulate between mosquitoes, non-human primates (chimpanzees, monkeys and baboons) and other vertebrate reservoirs like rodents and bats. The mosquitoes involved mainly inhabit the forests and include *Aedes* mosquitoes like: *Ae. luteocephalus, Ae. africanus, Ae. furcifer-taylori, Ae. dalzieli* and non-*Aedes* mosquitoes (*Culex, Mansonia),* among other mosquito species (Thiboutot et al., 2010).

It is speculated that one of the mosquito species that inhabited the forest, *Ae. aegypti formosus* had to adapt to survive, it therefore moved from the forest and started breeding and inhabiting storage containers near homesteads especially in urban settings and this led to the evolution and emergence of the *Ae. aegypti aegypti* phenotype (Powell et al., 2013). This corroborates the fact that CHIKV most likely emerged from the forests in Central Africa and spread to urban settings or near households and established the urban cycle. Mosquitoes like *Ae. aegypti* have been detected in African and in Asian urban settings (Diallo et al., 1999).

Outside of epidemics, CHIKV circulates in monkeys, rodents, birds, and other unidentified vertebrates, and in *Aedes* mosquitoes, principally *Ae. furcifer* and *Ae. africanus* which are found in the forested areas (Powers et al., 2000). In Senegal, through virus isolation, a number of CHIKV isolates were obtained from different endemic species of mosquitoes namely *Ae. luteocephalus, Ae. furcifer*, *Ae. africanus, Ae. taylori*, and *Ae. neoafricanus* (Diallo et al., 1999).

Urban Cycle of Chikungunya Virus

In Asia and urban settings, transmission and dissemination of CHIKV occurs between human and *Aedes species* of mosquitoes namely *Ae. aegypti,* and *Ae. albopictus* mosquitoes (Myers et al., 1965; Reuben, 1967). These two mosquito species can also transfer and spread other diseases, like Dengue, Zika, Yellow fever, Mayaro and are active during the day, hence, protective measures should be taken throughout the day. These two mosquito species are known to bite human outside the house, but *Ae. aegypti* readily bites even inside the houses. *Aedes aegypti,* and *Ae. albopictus* mosquitoes also readily breed in water stored around man-made containers around human households. Their adaptation to domestic and urban settings, makes it easy for them to infect humans.

In 1894 in India, *Ae. albopictus* mosquito, was identified and its enzootic to Southeast Asia. *Aedes albopictus* mosquitoes has spread to many countries through international travel and trade and it has been established in both temperate and tropical countries (Lounibos, 2002). *Aedes aegypti* flourishes during epidemics because of its behaviour and ecology that makes it prefer getting a blood meal from human rather than other animals. During the period between a blood meal and oviposition, the adult female mosquitoes feed on many blood meals and prefer man-made containers as larval breeding sites (Gubler, 2002).

During and after outbreaks, laboratory confirmed cases of Chikungunya and associated fatalities are usually reported. In Some instances, the vector involved in virus transmission is also documented. Below we shall explore some studies of mosquito species that were involved in certain outbreaks.

During the Chikungunya outbreak in the Reunion Island in 2006, CHIKV was mainly transmitted via *Ae. albopictus,* after a mutation (E1: A226V) which occurred in this CHIKV strain (Tsetsarkin et al., 2007). This genetic change in Reunion Island, was a substitution of a single amino acid from an Alanine to Valine at the E1 glycoprotein in amino acid position 226. The reported outbreaks in 2005 in Kenya, Seychelles and Comoros Island identified *Ae. aegypti* as the responsible vector that caused the viral disease to spread.

During the Chikungunya outbreak in Comoros, surveys of larvae showed diverse species of mosquitoes inhabited the Island. These included competent vectors namely*: Ae. vittatus, Eretmapodites chrysogaster and* Ae. *aegypti* among other mosquito species (Sang et al., 2008 and Mangiafico, 1971). Earlier reports showed that imported travelers from East African countries or Indian Ocean Islands arriving in India, were infected with Chikungunya, which may have been transmitted and spread by *Ae. aegypti* mosquitoes (Sudeep and Parashar, 2008).

Arrival of asymptomatic patient in Italy in 2007, who become symptomatic after a few days, caused a great concern and fear of a Chikungunya outbreak in Europe. Further laboratory analysis demonstrated that of *Ae. albopictus* was responsible for local transmission in Italy around the time the index patient arrived (Bordi et al., 2008).

In 2006, Sri-Lanka reported an enormous Chikungunya outbreak and most of the cases that were reported were mainly from the coastal and urban setting towns, however later on in 2008, cases were more common in plantation areas and were transmitted by *Ae. albopictus* (Hapuarachchi et al., 2010).

In a study conducted in Singapore, a number of adult mosquitoes namely *Culex quinquefasciatus and Ae. albopictus* were collected. To detect CHIKV in the mosquito homogenates, Reverse Transcription-Polymerase Chain Reaction (RT-PCR) was done and during the pre-intervention period, approximately 8.4% of the adult female mosquitoes (*Ae. albopictus)* tested positive for the virus (Tan et al., 2011).

In 2016, the Chikungunya outbreak that was reported in Mandera, located in Northeastern Kenya, had mosquitoes breeding in containers that were used for water storage both indoors and outdoors and the mosquitoes responsible for transmission and dissemination of this virus was *Ae. aegypti* (Konongoi et al., 2018).

A possible vertical transmission of *Ae. aegypti* in India, provided a reasonable way for the virus to survive in between epidemics (Rampal et al., 2007). During an entomological study in Kelantan, Malaysia, various containers were inspected to find out the breeding sites of *Aedes* mosquitoes. It was found that 97 containers had *Ae. albopictus* and tested positive for CHIKV.

Alternative Transmission Pathways

Chikungunya virus is generally maintained between humans, mosquitoes and other reseirvoir hosts. Other modes of transmission include vertical transmission, which is the transfer of virus from mother to feotus/child during pregnancy or at birth, respectively. Mother to child infection that is acquired towards the end of gestation, have resulted in symptomatic neonates with CHIKV infection. These infected neonates presented with fever, difficulty in feeding, and irritability after 3 to 9 days. Sometimes in cases where the mother gets infected with Chikungunya during early gestation periods, feotuses have been lost (Torres et al., 2016). Virus transfer through infected fluids like blood and organs is also hypothetically feasible during the outbreak, although no infections of this kind have been reported (Burt et al., 2012). So far reports of virus transmission from one human to another has not been documented.

Transmission of CHIKV through blood meal as mosquito feeds and transfers its saliva to human is the common mode of virus dissemination and vertical transmission can also occur through infected eggs. To mimic CHIKV vector infection, mosquitoes from endemic locations can be bred in a laboratory insectary, and fed on artificial blood meals infected with standard virus titres. The Mosquitoes are fed on CHIKV infected blood meal and, are kept in an insectary with controlled temperature and humidity for a number of days depending on the virus, in this case at least 7 days and then viral transmission is monitored. The infected mosquito disseminates the virus from the midgut to the hemocoel. Transmission potential is measured by the presence of CHIKV in the saliva and is used to infer the ability of the mosquitoes to disseminate the virus.

The capability of these mosquitoes to successfully disseminate the virus to another host is determined by a number of factors. Climate change can affect transmission rates of virus by determining the geographic spread and abundance of the mosquito vector. High temperature may cause mosquitos to endure but still increase their numbers in the population, alter their seasons, latitudes and altitudes as vectors thrive. Other factors that affect virus transmission include: vector population densities, abundance and availability of susceptible hosts and efficiency of viral replication (Coffey et al., 2014 and Zouache et al., 2014). Use of sylvatic or urban transmission cycles depends on availability of mosquito vector, hosts and the type of habitat.

Reservoirs of Chikungunya Virus

Reservoir of a pathogen is the natural environment where causative agent exists, breeds and flourish. Examples of reservoirs are animals, humans and birds.

Arboviruses circulate in interspersed transmission cycles between animal reservoir hosts and mosquito vectors, which poses a great risk of spillover of the virus into human populations. The spillover of arboviruses into humans can occur in 2 ways. One way is dissemination from a reservoir host species to humans. Alternatively, it can occur in two steps from the reservoir to an amplification host species and then to humans. Many reservoir host species in a particular environment may exchange an arbovirus among themselves and result in a reservoir community. After creation of a pool of viruses, endemic arboviruses can spillover and spread to humans in one-step from the reservoir community to the human host.

On the other hand, transmission of an arbovirus may occur from a reservoir host to diverse amplification hosts that are able to replicate efficiently, but may not be good for the long-term persistence of the virus. In this case, the virus spills-over to the human host directly from the amplifying host (Weaver, 2005 and Vorou et al., 2016).

Other Possible Reservoir Hosts

During an experimental set-up where animal models are to be used, a number of factors are considered. The animal should be susceptible and responsive to the specific virus, facilitate its replication and also exhibit specific clinical signs of viral infection which can be observed for modification in the presence of the antiviral compound. Depending on the animal species, the clinical signs should include histopathological changes, emaciation, lethargy and virus recovery from tissues. These animal models must also represent humans, in terms of clinical signs, histopathological changes, virus replication and growth kinetics (Bouvier and Lowen, 2010).

Many studies have been done to assess the susceptibility of different animal models to CHIKV in case of exposure to this virus and eventual transmission to another host or human. Arboviruses isolated from the forest-dwelling mosquitoes sometimes spread to human and domestic animals. Some of these hosts like rodents, some non-human primates and wildlife may be secondary hosts, but not critical for the persistence of the virus. On the other hand, these hosts can accommodate and nourish many arboviruses, making them significant hosts in zoonotic cycles. (Davis et al., 2005 and Jackson et al., 2015). Evidence also shows that wild non-human primates like monkeys can serve as pools of virus outside outbreaks (Osterrieth et al., 1960).

In Democratic Republic of Congo, chimpanzees were exposed to CHIKV and produced detectable neutralizing antibodies, while in Southern Africa, these antibodies were also detected from vervet monkeys, and chacma baboons (McIntosh et al., 1964 and Osterrieth et al., 1960). Primates which included gorillas, baboons and, chimpanzees, among other animals tested positive for CHIKV specific antibodies soon after arrival in the United States from Africa (Harrison et al., 1967).

Chikungunya virus specific antibodies were also reported in 10% of Patas monkeys, 7% of Tantalus monkeys, and 20% of Mona monkeys in Nigeria (Boorman and Draper, 1968).

Circulation of CHIKV in mosquitoes like *Ae. africanus that* prefer blood meal from animals have been reported in Uganda and in Asian countries like Malaysia and Thailand, CHIKV specific antibodies were also identified in non-human primates (McCrae et al., 1971 and Marchette et al., 1978).

Experimental studies in wild African rodents species (genera *Arcicanthis* and *Aethomys) and bats* got exposed to CHIKV and developed low viral loads, while other rodents (*Mystromys* species) developed a high viral load and at the same time, CHIKV specific neutralizing antibodies could be detected from their sera (Bosco-Lauth et al., 2016).

Chikungunya virus is a zoonotic disease and the susceptibility of domestic animals like sheep, goats, pigs, cattle, pigs, dogs, rabbits and horses to this virus should be a public health concern because studies in domestic animals show that they do not produce detectable viremia on virus exposure, but they have developed detectable CHIKV specific neutralizing antibodies (Halstead et al., 1966). These domestic animals need to be monitored closely and their vireamia status checked routinely.

CONCLUSION

Chikungunya outbreaks have emerged in the last century with outbreaks being reported across the globe and cases being detected in almost every continent. The spread of this virus is mainly facilitated by the distribution and abundance of the mosquito vector in different regions. Climatic conditions like temperature and humidity may favour mosquito breeding and their abundance. This would then determine whether the virus thrives in the tropical or temperate countries. As the virus spreads and adapts to different mosquito species during outbreaks, mutations have occurred leading to emerging strains of CHIKV. These mutations have the capacity to facilitate and enhance transmission of virus. For these reasons, more studies need to be done to clearly elucidate the possible reservoir hosts, vector abundance and distribution and how they interact in natural environment.

REFERENCES

AbuBakar, S., Sam, I. C., Wong, P. F., MatRahim, N. A., Hooi, P. S. and Roslan, N. 2007. "Reemergence of endemic Chikungunya, Malaysia." *Emerging Infectious Diseases* 13:147–149.

Arankalle, V. A., Shrivastava, S., Cherian, R. S., Gunjikar, A. M., Walimbe, S. M., Jadhav, A. B., Sundeep, A. C. and Mishra, 2007. "Genetic divergence of Chikungunya viruses in India (1963-2006) with special reference to the 2005-2006 explosive epidemic." *Journal of General Virology* 88:1967-1976.

Boorman, J. P. T., Draper, C. C. 1968. "Isolations of arboviruses in the Lagos area of Nigeria, and a survey of antibodies to them in man and animals." *Transactions of Royal Society of Tropical Medicine and Hygiene* 62: 269-277.

Bordi, L, Carletti, F, Castilletti, C, Chiappini, R, Sambri, V, Cavrini, F, et al. 2008. "Presence of the A226 V mutation in autochthonous and imported Italian chikungunya virus strains." *Clinical Infectious Disease* 47:428–429.

Bosco-Lauth, A. M., Nemeth, N. M., Kohler, D. J. and Bowen, R. A. 2016. "Viremia in North American mammals and birds after experimental infection with chikungunya viruses." *American Journal of Tropical Medicine and Hygiene* 94, 504–506.

Bouvier, Nicole M. and Lowen, Anice C. 2010. "Animal Models for Influenza Virus Pathogenesis and Transmission." *Viruses* 2, no. 8: 1530-1563.

Burt, F. J., Rolph, M. S., Rulli, N. E., Mahalingam, S., Heise, M. T. 2012. "Chikungunya: a re-emerging virus". *Lancet* 379 no. 9816: 662–71.

Carey, D. E. 1971. "Chikungunya and dengue: a case of mistaken identity? " *Journal of the History of Medicine and Allied Sciences* 26: 243-262.

Coffey, L. L., Failloux, A. B., Weaver, S. C. 2014. "Chikungunya virus–vector interactions." *Viruses 6*: 4628-4663.

Davis, S., Valvet, E., Leris, H. 2005. "Fluctuating rodent populations and risk to humans from rodent-borne zoonoses." *Vector Borne Zoonotic Dis*eases 5: 305-314.

Diallo, M., Thonnon, J., Traore-Lamizana, M. and Fontenille, D. 1999. "Vectors of Chikungunya virus in Senegal: current data and transmission cycles". *American Journal of Tropical Medicine and Hygiene* 60: 281–286.

Dupont-Rouzeyrol, M., Caro, V., Guillaumot, L., Vazeille, M., D' Ortenzio, E., Thiberge, J. M., Baroux, N., Gourinat, A. C., Grandadam, M. and Failloux, A. B. 2012. "Chikungunya virus and the mosquito vector *Aedes aegypti* in New Caledonia (South Pacific Region)." *Vector Borne Zoonotic Diseases* 12:1036-41.

Geser, A., Henderson, B. E. and Christensen, S. 1970. "A multipurpose serological survey in Kenya: 2. Results of arbovirus serological tests." *Bulletin of the World Health Organization* 43(4), 539-552.

Griffin, D. 2001. Alphaviruses. In: Knipe DM, Howley PM, editors. *Fields virology*. Philadelphia: Lippincott Williams & Wilkins. pp 917–962.

Gubler, D. J. 2002. “Epidemic Dengue/Dengue hemorrhagic fever as a public health, social and economic problem in the 21st century.” *Trends in Microbiology* 10: 100-103.

Gubler, D. J. 2011. “Dengue, Urbanization and Globalization: The Unholy Trinity of the 21(st) Century.” *Tropical Medicine and Health* 39: 3–11

Halstead, S. B. 1966. “Mosquito-borne haemorrhagic fevers of South and South-East Asia.” *Bulletin of the World Health Organization 35*: 3.

Hapuarachchi, H. A., Bandara K. B., Hapugoda M. D, Williams D. and Abeyewickreme W. 2008. “Laboratory confirmation of dengue and Chikungunya co-infection.” *Ceylon Medicine Journal* 53,104-105.

Hapuarachchi, H. C., Bandara, K. B., Sumanadasa, S. D., Hapugoda, M. D., Lai, Y. L., Lee, K. S., et al. 2010. “Re-emergence of Chikungunya virus in South-east Asia: virological evidence from Sri Lanka and Singapore.” *Journal of General Virology* 91:1067–76.

Harrison, V. R., Binn, L. N., Randall, R. 1967. “Comparative Immunogenicities of Chikungunya vaccines prepared in avian and mammalian tissues.” *American Journal of Tropical Medicine and Hygiene* 16: 786-91.

Horwood, P. F., Reimer, L. J., Dagina, R., Susapu, M., Bande, G., Katusele, M., Koimbu, G., Jimmy, S., Ropa, B., Siba, P. M. and Pavlin, B. I. 2013. “Outbreak of Chikungunya virus infection, vanimo, Papua New Guinea.” *Emerging Infectious Diseases* 19, no. 9: 1535-1538.

Jackson, J. A. 2015. “Immunology in wild non-model rodents: an ecological context for studies of health and disease.” *Parasite Immunology* 37:220–32.

Kariuki, N. M., Nderitu, L., Ledermann, J. P., Ndirangu, A., Logue, C. H., Kelly, C. H., Sang, R., Sergon, K., Breiman, R. and Powers, A. M. 2008. “Tracking epidemic Chikungunya virus into the Indian Ocean from East Africa.” *Journal of General Virology* 89:2754–2760.

Khongwichit, S., , Jira Chansaenroj, Thanunrat Thongmee, Saovanee Benjamanukul, Nasamon Wanlapakorn, Chintana Chirathaworn, Yong Poovorawa. 2021. “Large-scale outbreak of Chikungunya virus infection in Thailand 2018–2019: March 10, 2021, doi.org/10.1371/journal.pone.0247314.

Konongoi, S.L., Nyunja, A., Ofula, V., Owaka, S., Koka, H., Koskei, E, et al. 2018. "Human and entomologic investigations of chikungunya outbreak in Mandera, Northeastern Kenya, 2016." *PLoS ONE* 13 no. 10: e0205058.

Lanciotti, R. S., Kosoy, O. L., Laven, J. J., Panella, A. J., Velez, J. O., Lambert, A. J. and Campbell, G. L. 2007. "Chikungunya virus in US travelers returning from India, 2006." *Emerging Infectious Diseases* 13: 764-77.

Laras, K., Sukri, N. C., Larasati, R. P., Bangs, M. J., Kosim, R., Djauzi, Wandra T., Master, J., Kosasih, H., Hartati, S., Beckett, C., Sedyaningsih, E. R., Beecham, H. J. and Corwin, A. L. 2005. "Tracking the re-emergence of epidemic Chikungunya virus in Indonesia." *Transactions of the Royal Society of Tropical Medicine and Hygiene* 99:128–141.

Leo, Y. S., Chow, A. L. P., Tan, L. K., Lye, D. C., Lin, L. and Ng, L. C. 2009. "Chikungunya outbreak, Singapore, 2008." *Emerging Infectious Diseases* 15, 836–837.

Leparc-Goffart, I., Nougairede, A., Cassadou, S., Prat, C. and de Lamballerie, X. 2014. "Chikungunya in the Americas, correspondence." *Lancet* 383:514.

Lounibos, L. P. 2002. "Invasions by insect vectors of human disease." *Annual Review of Entomology* 47: 233-266.

Lumsden, W. H. 1955. "An epidemic of virus disease in Southern Province, Tanganyika Territory, in 1952-53. II. General description and epidemiology". *Transactions of the Royal Society of Tropical Medicine and Hygiene* 49: 33-57.

Lutomiah, J., Bast, J., Clark, J., Richardson, J., Yalwala, S., Oullo, D., Mutisya, J., Mulwa, F., Musila, L, Khamadi, S., Schnabel, D., Wurapa, E. and Sang, R. 2013. "Abundance, diversity, and distribution of mosquito vectors in selected ecological regions of Kenya: public health implications." *Journal of Vector Ecology* 38:134-42.

Mangiafico, J. A. 1971. "Chikungunya virus infection and transmission in five species of mosquito." *American Journal of Tropical Medicine and Hygiene* 20:642–645.

Marchette, N. J., Rudnick, A., Garcia, R., Mac Vean, S. 1978. "Alphaviruses in Peninsular Malaysia. I. Virus isolations and animal serology. "Southeast *Asian Journal of Tropical Medicine and Public Health* 9: 317- 29.

McCrae, A. W. R., Henderson, B. E., Kirya, B. G. & Sempala, S. D. K. 1971. "Chikungunya virus in the Entebbe area of Uganda: isolations and epidemiology." *Transactions of the Royal Society Tropical Medicine and Hygiene* 65:152–168.

McIntosh, B. M., Paterson, H. E., McGillivray, G., De Sousa, J. 1964. "Further Studies on the Chikungunya Outbreak in Southern Rhodesia in 1962: I.—Mosquitoes, Wild Primates and Birds in Relation to the Epidemic." *Annals of Tropical Medicine & Parasitology* 58: 45-51.

Mease, L., Coldren, R. L., Musila, L. A., Prosser, T., Ogolla, F., Ofula, V. O., Schoepp, R. J., Rossi, C. A. and Adungo, N. 2011. "Seroprevalence and distribution of arboviral infections among rural Kenyan adults, a cross-sectional study." *Virology Journal* 27, no.8: 371-379.

Morrill, J., Johnson, B., Hyams, C., Okoth, F., Tukei, P., Mugambi, M. and Woody, J. 1991. "Serological evidence of arboviral infections among humans of coastal Kenya." *Journal of Tropical Medicine and Hygiene* 94:166-168.

Mwongula, A. W., Mwamburi, L. A., Matilu, M., Siamba, D. N. and Wanyama, F. W. 2013. "Seroprevalence of Chikungunya Infection in Pyretic Children Seeking Treatment in Alupe District Hospital, Busia County Kenya". *International Journal of Current Microbiology and Applied Sciences* 2 no. 5: 130-139.

Myers, R. M., Carey, D. E., Reuben, R., Jesudass E. S., de Ranitz C. D., Jadhav M. 1965. "The 1964 epidemic of dengue-like fever in South India: isolation of Chikungunya virus from human sera and from mosquitoes." *Indian Journal of Medical Research* 53:694–701.

Osterrieth, P., and Blanes-Ridaura G. 1960. "Research on the Chikungunya virus in the Belgian Congo. I. Isolation of the virus in upper Uele."

Annales de la Societe belge de medecine tropicale (1920), 40,199-203. [*Annals of the Belgian Society of Tropical Medicine*]

Powers, A. and Logue, C. 2007. "Changing patterns of Chikungunya virus: re-emergence of a zoonotic arbovirus." *Journal of General Virology* 88: 2363- 2377.

Powers, A. M. 2011. "Genomic evolution and phenotypic dinstinctions of Chikungunya viruses causing the Indian Ocean outbreak." *Experimental Biology and Medicine* 236:909-914.

Powers, A. M., Brault, A. C., Tesh, R. B. and Weaver, S. C. 2000. "Re-emergence of Chikungunya and O'nyong - nyong viruses: Evidence for distinct geographical lineages and distant evolutionary relationships." *Journal of General Virology* 81:471-479.

Rampal, Sharda M., Meena H. 2007. "Hypokalemic paralysis following Chikungunya fever." *Journal of the Association of Physicians of India* 55:598.

Ravi, V. 2006. "Re-emergence of Chikungunya virus in India." *Indian Journal of Medical Microbiology* 24, 83-84.

Renault, P., Solet, J. L., Sissoko, D., Balleydier, E., Larrieu, S., Filleul, L., Lassalle, C., Thiria, J., Rachou, E., De Valk, H., Ilef, D., Ledrans, M., Quatresous, I., Quenel, P. and Pierre, V. 2007. "A major epidemic of Chikungunya virus infection in Reunion Island, France, 2005-2006." *American Journal of Tropical Medicine and Hygiene* 77, no. 4: 727-731.

Reuben, R. 1967. "Some entomological and epidemiological observations on the 1964 outbreak of Chikungunya fever in South India." *Indian Journal of Medical Research 55:1*–12.

Rezza, G., Nicoletti, L., Angelini, R., Romi, R., Finarelli, A. C., Panning, M., Cordioli, P., Fortuna, C., Boros, S., Magurano, F., Silvi, G., Angelini, P., Dottori, M., Ciufolini, M. G., Majori, G. C. and Cassone, A. 2007. "Infection with Chikungunya virus in Italy: an outbreak in a temperate region." *Lancet 370*, no. 9602 1840-1846.

Robinson, M. C. 1955. "An epidemic of virus disease in Southern Province, Tanganyika Territory, in 1952–1953 I. Clinical features." *Transactions of the Royal Society of Tropical Medicine and Hyg*iene 49:28–32.

Ross, R. W. 1956. "The Newala epidemic. III. The virus: isolation, pathogenic properties and relationship to the epidemic. "*Journal of Hygiene (London)* 54: 177-191.

Sang, R. C., Ahmed, O., Faye, O., Kelly, C. L., Yahaya, A. A., Mmadi, I., Toilibou, A. Sergon, K., Brown, J., Agata, N., Yakouide, A., Ball, M. D., Breiman, R. F., Miller, B. R. and Powers, A. M. 2008. "Entomologic investigations of a Chikungunya virus epidemic in the Union of the Comoros, 2005." *American Journal of Tropical Medicine and Hygiene* 78:77–82.

Schuffenecker, I., Iteman, I., Michault, A., Murri, S., Frangeul, L., Vaney, M. C., Lavenir, R., Pardigon, N., Reynes, J. M., Pettinelli, F., Biscornet, L., Diancourt, L., Michel, S., Duquerroy, S., Guigon, G., Frienkiel, M. P., Brehin, A. C., Cubito, N., Despres, P., Kunst, F., Rey, F. A., Zeller, H. and Brisse, S. 2006. "Genome microevolution of Chikungunya viruses causing the Indian Ocean outbreak." *PLoS Medicine* 3, e263.

Sergon, K., Njuguna, C., Kalani, R., Ofula, V., Onyango, C., Konongoi, L. S., Bedno, S., Burke H., Dumilla, A. M., Konde, J., Njenga, M. K., Sang, R. and Breiman, R. F. 2008. "Seroprevalence of Chikungunya virus (CHIKV) infection on Lamu Island, Kenya, October 2004." *American Journal of Tropical Medicine and Hygiene* 78:333–337.

Sergon, K., Yahaya, A. A., Brown, J., Bedja, S. A., Mlindasse, M., Agata, N., Allaranger, Y., Ball, M. D., Powers, A. M., Ofula, V., Onyango, C., Konongoi, L. S., Sang, R., Njenga, M. K. and Breiman, R. F. 2007. "Seroprevalence of Chikungunya virus infection on Grande Comore Island, Union of the Comoros, March 2005." *American Journal of Tropical Medicine and Hygiene* 76: 1189–1193.

Sudeep, A. B., Parashar, D. 2008. "Chikungunya: an overview." *Journal of Biosciences* 33:443–9.

Sutherland, L. J., Cash, A. A., Huang, Y. J S., Sang, R. C., Malhotra, I., Moormann, A. M., King, C. L., Weaver, S. C., King, C. H. and LaBeaud, D. 2011. "Serologic evidence of arboviral infections among humans in Kenya." *American Journal of Tropical Medicine and Hygiene* 85, no. 1:158 -161.

Tan, C. H., Wong, P. S., Li, M. Z., Tan, S. Y., Lee, T. K., Pang, S. C., Lam-Phua, S. G., Maideen, N., Png, A. B., Koou, S. Y., Lu, D., and Ng, L. C. 2011. "Entomological investigation and control of a chikungunya cluster in Singapore". *Vector borne and zoonotic diseases (Larchmont, N. Y.) 11, no.* 4: 383–390.

Theamboonlers, A., Rianthavorn, P., Praianantathavom, K., Wuttirattanakowit, N. and Poovorawan, Y. 2009. "Clinical and molecular characterization of Chikungunya virus in South Thailand." *Japanese Journal of Infectious Diseases* 62: 303-305.

Thiboutot, M. M., Kannan, S., Kawalekar, O. U., Shedlock, D. J., Khan, A. S., Sarangan, G., Srikanth, P., Weiner, D. B. and Muthumani, K. 2010. "Chikungunya: a potentially emerging epidemic?" *PLoS Neglected Tropical Diseases 4* no. 4: e623.

Torres, J. R., Falleiros-Arlant, L. H., Dueñas, L., Pleitez-Navarrete, J., Doris M. Salgado, D. M. and José Brea-Del Castillo. 2016. "Congenital and perinatal complications of chikungunya fever: a Latin American experience." *International Journal of Infectious Diseases* 51:85–88.

Tsetsarkin, K. A., Vanlandingham, D. L., McGee, C. E. and Higgs, S. 2007. "A single mutation in Chikungunya virus affects vector specificity and epidemic potential." *PLoS Pathogens* 3, e201.

Vorou, R. 2016. "Zika virus, vectors, reservoirs, amplifying hosts, and their potential to spread worldwide: what we know and what we should investigate urgently." *International Journal of Infectious Disease*. 48, 85–90.

Warner, E., Garcia-Diaz, J., Balsamo, G., Shranatan, S., Bergmann, A., Blauwet, L., Sohail, M., Baddour, L. and Reed, C. 2006. "Chikungunya fever diagnosed among international travelers – United States, 2005–2006." *Morbidity and Mortality Weekly Report* 55: 1040–1042.

Wasonga, C., Inoue, S., Kimotho, J., Morita, K., Ongus, J., Sang, R. and Musila, L. 2015. "Development and Evaluation of an in-house IgM ELISA for the Detection of Chikungunya and Application to a Dengue Outbreak Situation in Kenya in 2013." *Japanese Journal of Infectious Diseases* 68 no. 5: 410-414.

Weaver, S. C. 2005. "Host range, amplification and arboviral disease emergence. (In: Peters, C. J., and Calisher, C. H.)" *Infectious Diseases from Nature, Mechanisms of Viral Emergence and Persistence.* 33–44 Springer, Vienna. https://doi.org/10.1007/3-211-29981-5_4.

Weaver, S. C. and Reisen, W. K. 2009. "Present and future arboviral threats." *Antiviral Research* 85:328–345.

Wu, D., Zhang, Y., Zhouhui, Q., Kou, L., Liang, W., Zhang, H., Monagin, C., Zhang, Q., Li W., Zhong, H., He, J., Li, H., Cai, S., Ke, C. and Lin, J. 2013. "Chikungunya virus with E1-A226V mutation causing causing two outbreaks in 2010, Guangdong, China" *Virology Journal* 10:174.

Yoosuf, A. A., Shiham, I., Mohamed, A. J., Ali, G., Luna, J. M., Pandav, R., Gongal, G. N., Nisaluk, A., Jarman, R. G. and Gibbons, R. V. 2008. "First report of Chikungunya from the Maldives." *Transactions of the Royal Society of Tropical Medicine and Hygiene* 103 no. 2: 192-196.

Zouache, K., Fontaine, A., Vega-Rua, A., Mousson, L., Thiberge, J. M., Lourenco-De-Oliveira, R., Failloux, A. B. 2014. "Three-way interactions between mosquito population, viral strain and temperature underlying chikungunya virus transmission potential." *Proceedings of the Royal Society of London: Biological Sciences* 281 no. 1792: 20141078

In: Chikungunya
Editor: Phillip Galvan

ISBN: 978-1-53619-978-9

Chapter 3

RECENT PROGRESS ON IMMUNOTHERAPY AND IMMUNOPROPHYLAXIS OF CHIKUNGUNYA VIRUS

Himanshu Sehrawat[1], Mohd Fardeen Husain Shahanshah[1], Chanuka Wijewardana[1], Sachin Pal[1], Vijay K. Chaudhary[2], Sanjay Gupta[3] and Vandana Gupta[1,*]

[1]Department of Microbiology, Ram Lal Anand College, University of Delhi, Benito Juarez Road, New Delhi, India
[2]Centre for Innovation in Infectious Disease Research, Education and Training, University of Delhi South Campus, Benito Juarez Marg, India
[3]Centre for Emerging Diseases, Department of Biotechnology, Jaypee Institute of Information Technology, Noida, India

[*] Corresponding Author's E-mail: vandanagupta72@rediffmail.com; vandanagupta@rla.du.ac.in.

Abstract

The resurging CHIKV outbreaks and epidemics have presented several socio-economic challenges to the world. Even after 60 years of its discovery, there are still no approved therapies or vaccines. The scientific community today is in pursuit of rapid development of antivirals and prophylactics. In this chapter, we provide an insight into the different Immunotherapy and Immunoprophylaxis strategies that have demonstrated promising results so far and are under development and others that are developed and approved for CHIKV.

Abbreviations

CHIKV	Chikungunya virus
CHIKF	Chikungunya fever
nsP	nonstructural proteins
IFN:	Interferon
NSAID	Non-steroidal anti-inflammatory drugs
MV	Measles Virus
mAbs	Monoclonal Antibodies
nAbs	Neutralizing Antibodies
Abs	Antibodies

Introduction

Chikungunya fever (CHIKF) is an arthropod borne viral illness. Infected *Aedes* mosquito transmits CHIKV or Chikungunya virus to humans while feeding on them. It leads to severe morbidity in patients through inflammation of the musculoskeletal system. The identified causal agent is an RNA virus classified under the family Togaviridae. This alphavirus possesses a single-stranded, non-segmented, positive-sense RNA genome encapsidated in an icosahedral capsid which is tightly associated with a host-derived lipid bilayer envelope (Rupp et al., 2015). CHIKV manifests a range of signs and symptoms with profound myalgia and polyarthralgia. Along with these, the patient may also suffer from high fever, headache, rigors, and maculopapular rashes (Silva & Dermody 2017; Schwartz and Albert 2010; Weaver and Lecuit 2015, Hucke and Bugert 2020). Till 2004, this disease was largely confined to the tropics of Southeast Asia, South America, and Central Africa but now reach of this pathogen has expanded probably due to the abrupt climate changes that led to the expansion of habitat of its vector/s (*Aedes aegypti* and *Aedes albopictus*) (Schwartz and Albert 2010; Pérez-Pérez et al., 2019; Hucke and Bugert 2020).

CHIKV has caused recurring outbreaks in over 40 countries of the world and became endemic to even temperate territories of Southern Europe, Northern Asia, and Northern America (Schwartz and Albert 2010; Pérez-Pérez et al., 2019; Hucke and Bugert 2020).

The epidemiological burden of the disease can be mitigated by encouraging research and the development of efficacious therapeutics and potent vaccines. Over the last few decades, several promising vaccine candidates and monoclonal antibodies have been developed against CHIKV. However, none of them have been approved for clinical use. This chapter gives the reader a comprehensive overview of the same.

PASSIVE IMMUNIZATION OR IMMUNO-THERAPEUTIC APPROACH TO CHIKV

Passive immunization achieved by the administration of antibodies provides transient protection from the disease in the already infected individuals. Antibodies serve as effector molecules of humoral immunity and neutralize antigens by specifically binding to them and marking them for elimination (Kindt TJ 2007). Antibodies could provide antiviral effects via antibody-mediated phagocytosis, antibody-dependent cytotoxicity, and complement-dependent cytotoxicity, which may directly destroy the virus or/and the virus-infected cells. As the administration of preformed antibodies in the patient generates a rapid response, they are employed as immuno-therapeutics. Based on this knowledge, several types of immunotherapies against CHIKV have been articulated.

Convalescent Plasma Therapy

Generally, individuals who have recovered from infectious disease have high titers of neutralizing antibodies that are specific to the causal agent. Convalescent plasma can be administered to patients who have acquired the same infection to alleviate their symptoms and chances of mortality. The use of passive immunization therapy using convalescent plasma can be traced back to the 1890s. Convalescent Plasma therapy has been successfully used to treat several infectious diseases, particularly during a large-scale epidemic or pandemic due to the availability of patients' undergone convalescence willing to donate the plasma. Thus, convalescent plasma transfusion (CPT) has become the topic of increasing interest, especially in the wake of epidemics and pandemics as is evident in the current COVID-19 Pandemic (Kaur and Gupta 2020; Casadevall 2020; Singh and Gupta 2021). CPT as a modality of treatment for Chikungunya fever has been tested in mouse models and can be implemented during extensive outbreaks or epidemics (Couderc et al., 2009).

Monoclonal Antibodies

The use of monoclonal antibodies is a favored approach over CPT as a therapeutic option for CHIKV. Monoclonal Ab-based therapeutics also offers several advantages over vaccine-induced immunity. It provides immediate protection and is safe in high-risk populations in particular the elderly patients, immunocompromised individuals, and pregnant women. During emergencies, they can be transported and distributed more quickly than vaccines (Sparrow et al., 2017). Development and use of a highly specific Ab-based therapeutic regimen can alter the progress of an epidemic (Mavalankar et al., 2008). The administration of antibodies can elicit an instantaneous action whereas vaccines require a longer duration (from a few weeks to several months) to generate a protective immune response and therefore remain the therapeutics of choice under severe conditions (Freitas et al., 2018).

Antibody-based therapeutics have a higher success rate in viral diseases like CHIKV where the genome of the virus is comparatively conserved and does not undergo frequent mutations. CHIKV is highly conserved when compared to the other exceptionally variable viruses such as Hepatitis, HIV, and Influenza. The envelope protein sequence of different chikungunya virus lineages is highly conserved and hence can be considered as potential targets (Erasmus et al., 2016). Different serotypes of the virus can be targeted by designing neutralizing antibodies specific to the conserved epitopes. Monoclonal Abs function either by directly neutralizing the target antigen or by indirect effector mechanisms such as Ab-dependent cell-mediated cytotoxicity (ADCC), Ab-mediated phagocytosis, and complement-dependent cytotoxicity (CDC), etc., wherein, mAbs bind to virus and infected cells and help in their clearance from the body (Hey 2015).

Entry Neutralization by mAbs

Convalescent sera of CHIKV patients possess neutralizing antibodies that specifically target the E2 glycoprotein of the virus (Kam et al., 2012). E2 and E1 viral glycoproteins work together in a complementary fashion and support viral entry by binding to the host cell and encouraging fusion of the viral membrane with the acidified endosome membrane respectively (Akahata et al., 2010; Jin and Simmons 2019; Weber et al., 2017).

The mature E2 protein, prominently expressed on the viral surface has three immunoglobulin-like extracellular domains which are interconnected with a beta ribbon. The central position of the protein is occupied by domain A (N terminal domain), domain C is closest in proximity to the viral membrane with domain B located at the tip. These domains have been identified as the principal sites on the CHIKV surface that play a vital role in interaction with host cells. Latest studies have shown that CHIKV gains entry into the host cells via two separate mechanisms, one is glycosaminoglycans (GAGs) dependent in which domain B is involved and another is GAG-independent which engages domain A. Such investigations emphasize the importance of these two domains and their potential as promising targets for nAb based therapeutics (Weber et al., 2017). Several monoclonal antibodies targeting the domains of the E2 viral protein have been isolated, and their therapeutic efficacies have been tested in various animal models (Jin and Simmons 2019; Zhang et al., 2018).

Neutralizing Abs CHK-152 and 5M16 can effectively arrest CHIKV fusion with the plasma membrane. The supposed activity of the nAbs may be due to the cross-linking of the flexible domain B to the remaining viral surface that keeps the fusion loop unexposed and preventing viral entry into the host cell (Pal et al., 2013; Long et al., 2015; Smith et al., 2015).

Inhibition of Viral Budding by mAbs

In addition to inhibiting the virus entry into cells some antibodies like mouse nAbs CHK-265 and CHK-187 and human nAbs C9 and IM-CKV063 can also suppress virion release from CHIKV infected cells (Jin et al., 2015). Bivalent binding of nAbs to the CHIKV glycoproteins represses viral release from the infected cell. The glycoproteins that are expressed on the surface of an infected cell get recognized by these nAbs and induce coalescence of the glycoprotein, thus preventing the budding of the emerging virions. It is still unknown whether the epitopes of glycoproteins involved in this process are the same as the ones that are present in mature viruses. Hence, more studies are required to ascertain the epitopes that are participating in binding to nAb (Jin et al., 2015).

Antibody-Activated Effector Functions

Monoclonal Abs also perform a range of effector functions which are vital to immunity through their interactions with the Fc receptors (Bournazos et al., 2015). These innate immunity effector functions are complement activation, antibody-dependent cellular cytotoxicity (ADCC) involving NK cells mediated killing of infected cells and monocytes, macrophages and neutrophils mediated antibody-dependent cell-mediated phagocytosis (ADCP) of the infected cells and virions (Bournazos et al., 2015). Innate immune cells in humans are known to possess six classical Fc gamma receptors including FcγRI, FcγRIIa, FcγRIIb, FcγRIIc, FcγRIIIa, and FcγRIIIb. These are expressed in diverse combinations on all the cells involved in innate immune response at varying levels (Bruhns et al., 2012). Out of all the six FcγRs, the only inhibitory receptor is FcγRIIb. The pattern of expression of the FcγRs on the effector cells and the affinity of the Fc for the particular receptor determine the cellular outcome of IgG-FcγR interactions (Nimmerjahn et al., 2008). Classical FcγRs bind in the vicinity of the hinge region of IgG and activate tyrosine-based activation motifs (ITAM) present either in the cytoplasmic domain or on the common γ chain. These immunoreceptors cluster during activation, initiating signaling cascade which stimulates immune cells to exhibit effector functions (Lu et al., 2015; Radaev et al., 2001; Getahun et al., 2015).

Besides FcγRI, the other five FcγRs show a low affinity for IgG and thus cannot bind monomeric IgG (Bournazos et al., 2015). Through multi-valent, high avidity interactions, antigen-IgG complexes adequately engage and crosslink low-affinity FcγRs, ultimately leading to initiate signal from the oligomerized FcγRs (Goodridge et al., 2012; Sondermann et al., 2001). Neutralizing Abs IM-CKV063 and C9 induces coalescence of glycoprotein on the cell membrane of cells infected with CHIKV thereby inhibiting the budding of nascent virions (Jin et al., 2018). The dense layer of coalesced nAb-Glycoprotein complexes on the surface of chikungunya virus-infected cells presents multi-valent Fc to Fc gamma receptors in abundance and effectively stimulates ADCC from effector cells that express the triggering FcγRIIIa (Jin et al., 2018). This suggests that the bivalent binding of IgGs with the expressed glycoproteins contributes to a potent ADCC activation. An Fc-FcγR interaction on monocytes is required for the optimal therapeutic activity of mAbs against the chikungunya virus. Humanized mAbs CHK-152 and CHK-166 which belong to the human IgG1 subclass could promote virus clearance, and reduce cell infiltration and foot swelling in mice when administered on the 3rd-day post-infection (Fox et al., 2019).

Neutralizing IgM mAbs

The monoclonal antibodies described till now are all IgGs. In humans, 5% of the serum antibodies are IgMs while 75% are IgGs (Jin and Simmons

2019). 3E7b is a neutralizing IgM antibody that has been developed against CHIKV. This IgM mAb targets the N218 epitope present in the domain B of E2 protein. It neutralizes CHIKV entry into the host cell and has an IC50 of 4.5 ng/mL which is comparable to the most potent human neutralizing IgG, 5M16 which has an IC50 of 3.4 ng/mL (Long et al., 2015; Lam et al., 2015).

IgM being pentameric may cause efficient crosslinking and coalescing of glycoproteins expressed on the membrane of cells infected with CHIKV and thus strongly inhibit virus budding. IgM is also the most effective type of antibody in the activation complement cascade through the classical pathway (Pluschke et al., 1989). This paves way for more research on the use of neutralizing IgMs as a therapy against CHIKV.

Monoclonal Abs can be designed to target an epitope which is crucial for virus replication and pathogenesis and hence, any escaping mutation within the epitope will be fatal for the virus or decrease the viral pathogenesis. Under such conditions, treatment with a single monoclonal antibody can successfully protect the host (Jin et al., 2015). Another approach would be to administer a cocktail of mAbs which target different antigenic sites. Viral load in the patient increases rampantly during the acute phase of the infection, which enhances the odds of a resistance variant to emerge. A concoction of mAbs will limit the emergence of such resistant mutants and provide more efficient protection (Pal et al., 2013; Pal et al., 2014).

With the advent of technology, highly potent and broadly cross-reactive mAbs against CHIKV and the other alphaviruses are under development. Table 1 enlists the promising mAbs that have been synthesized to target CHIKV.

Table 1. Monoclonal antibodies developed against CHIKV

S. No.	mAb	Species	Antigenic sites	Demonstrated mode of action	References
1	2H1	Human	Envelope protein 2-Domain A	Entry neutralization	Smith et al., 2015
2	8G18	Human	Envelope protein 2-Domain A	Entry neutralization	Smith et al., 2015
3	3E23	Human	Envelope protein 2-Domain A	Entry neutralization	Smith et al., 2015
4	1O6	Human	Envelope protein 2-Domain A	Entry neutralization	Smith et al.,2015
5	4J21	Human	Envelope protein 2-Domain A, Domain B, Arch	Entry neutralization	Smith et al.,2015; Long et al.,2015
6	5M16	Human	Envelope protein 2-Domain A, Domain B, Arch	Entry neutralization	Smith et al.,2015; Long et al., 2015
7	CHK-152	Mouse	Envelope protein 2-Domain A, Domain B, Arch	Entry neutralization, ADCP	Pal et al.,2013; Sun et al.,2013
8	CHK-9	Mouse	Envelope protein 2-Domain A	Entry neutralization	Pal et al.,2013; Sun et al.,2013
9	CHK-265	Mouse	Envelope protein 2-Domain A, Domain B	Entry neutralization	Pal et al.,2013
10	CHK-187	Mouse	Envelope protein 2-Domain B	Inhibition of viral egress/exit, entry neutralization	Pal et al., 2013
11	CK47	Mouse	Envelope protein 1-Domain 3	Inhibition of viral egress/exit	Masrinoul et al., 2014
12	CHK-166	Mouse	Envelope protein 1-D2	Entry neutralization, ADCP	Porta et al., 2014
13	m242	Human	Envelope protein 2-Domain A	Entry neutralization	Sun et al., 2013
14	m10	Human	Envelope protein 2-Domain B	Entry neutralization	Sun et al., 2013
15	C9	Human	Envelope protein 2-Domain A, Domain B, Arch	Entry neutralization, ADCC, budding inhibition	Jin et al., 2018
16	8B10	Human	Envelope protein 2-Domain B, Domain A	Entry neutralization, budding inhibition	Porta et al., 2014
17	5F10	Human	Envelope protein 2-Domain B	Entry neutralization, budding inhibition	Porta et al., 2014
18	IM-CKV063	Human	Envelope protein 2-Domain A, Domain B, Arch	Entry neutralization, ADCC, budding inhibition	Jin et al., 2018

Immuno-Prophylaxis

Long-term immunity against a pathogen is acquired through active immunization. The adaptive immune response gets triggered on exposure to the infectious agent and immunologic memory is developed. Besides contracting the disease, the same can be achieved through vaccines. When an individual has been successfully immunized, any successive exposure to the same pathogen elicits a secondary immune response that effectively eliminates the pathogen and does not let the disease progress to severe form (Kindt TJ 2007).Diseases that once took millions of lives have been successfully eradicated and kept under check through vaccination. So far numerous vaccine candidates using all the different available vaccine development platforms have been advanced against CHIKV, out of which, only two managed to reach the clinical trials. The pros and cons of the different vaccine development platforms are reviewed extensively by Kaur and Gupta (2020).

Virus-Like Particle

One of the very few vaccine candidates to reach advanced development is Virus-like particle (VLP) based vaccines. The immunogenic component of the vaccine comes from the multiple protein genes of CHIKV that usually encodes E1, E2, and capsid (C) structural proteins. These genes are expressed using an expression vector that has been transfected into tissue culture. The serological cross-reactivity and high similarity between genotypically different strains of CHIKV suggest that any strain of CHIKV can be used to develop a potent vaccine that can protect CHIKV of all genotypes (Goo et al., 2016; Powers et al., 2000).

VRC-CHKVLP059-00-VP

VRC-CHKVLP059-00-VP is the first VLP based vaccine against Chikungunya to reach clinical trials. Akahata and colleagues designed VLPs derived from both a West African genotype strain (37997) and an ECSA genotype strain (OPY-1). The genes of C-E3-E2-6K/TF-E1 proteins were expressed in an expression vector based on cytomegalovirus CMV/R, which was cultured in the human embryonic kidney (HEK) 293 cells (Akahata et al., 2010). A strong nAb response was mounted against not only the homologous but also the heterologous strains when intramuscular injections of the 37997 VLPs were administered in BALB/c mice and Macaques (Akahata et al., 2010). This VLP based approach looked effective in animal models and was taken to the Phase 1 human clinical trial to assess its safety, through a dose-escalation format (Chang et al., 2014). No arthralgia, fever, or serious reactogenicities were reported from the initial trial. After the second dose, all subjects were found to have developed nAbs. The serum collected from the volunteers contained nAbs which were demonstrated to be cross-protective against chikungunya viral strains across all the genotypes giving strength to the idea that a vaccine developed by using any viral strain would protect against various strains across CHIKV genotypes (Goo et al., 2016; Tharmarajah et al., 2017). From the phase II clinical trial, it was reported that the CHIKV VLP vaccine is well tolerated and highly immunogenic among healthy adults and elicits no serious adverse events. Subjects received two intramuscular (IM) injections of the vaccine on Day 0 and Day 28 at a dose of 20 micrograms (mcg). As of now, Phase 3 trials are needed to assess its clinical efficacy (Chen et al., 2020; Clinical trial 2020).

A VLP is structurally similar to an infectious virus but lacks nucleic acid and is therefore non-infectious. The VLP approach is preferred because it is safe for use in immunocompromised individuals, pregnant females, etc. Production of such vaccines is easy and large stocks can be manufactured swiftly. However, functionally it is a "killed" vaccine there are some concerns about its low immunogenicity. To counter this problem, multiple rounds of immunizations may be conducted or different adjuvant strategies may be tried to provide long-term immunity (Tharmarajah et al., 2017). Though excessive use of adjuvants may subvert the vaccine's tolerability and enhance its reactogenicity, hence further investigations are required (Tharmarajah et al., 2017).

DNA Vaccines

DNA-based vaccines are one of the most extensively explored approaches against CHIKV and are summarized in the following sections.

Plasmid Vectors Containing CHIKV Proteins

The development of DNA vaccines against the Chikungunya virus began with the construction of several plasmid vectors bearing genes encoding each of its structural proteins important in eliciting protective immune response namely capsid, E2, and E1 (Muthumani et al., 2008). To broaden the cross-protective efficacy of the vaccine, these viral genes were not procured from any single strain but the consensus sequences of all the different strains. The *in-vitro* and *in-vivo* studies demonstrated an efficient expression and generation of productive immune responses (Mallilankaraman et al., 2011). The same was confirmed in non-human primates as well (Mallilankaraman et al., 2011). Both humoral and cell-mediated immune responses were generated. Furthermore, outbred immunized mice were protected from the disease even upon lethal challenge (Bao et al., 2013). Furthermore, when plasmid vectors with nsP2 sequence were also incorporated into the system, the effect of the envelope protein vaccine got enhanced (Bao et al., 2013).

Plasmid Vectors Containing Attenuated CHIKV Genome

DNA vaccines expressing attenuated forms of the CHIKV genome have also been developed. The CHIKV genome was attenuated by deleting either the entire 6k gene or portions of the gene encoding for nsP3 (Hallengärd et al., 2014). A single dose of this DNA vaccine generated strong T cell responses and produced high levels of nAb in mice and macaques. It imparted protection against both foot swelling and viremia. Furthermore, the developed nAbs could neutralize the heterologous strain of the Asian genotype to a level that was comparable to those elicited to the homologous strains of the virus (Roques et al., 2017).

Complete protection against challenge was demonstrated after the administration of this attenuated viral DNA vaccine, but low levels of viremia were still seen upon immunization suggesting active viral multiplication due to limited attenuation (Tretyakova et al., 2014).

Hidajat and co-workers proposed a novel vaccination approach based on immunization DNA (iDNA®) infectious clone technology wherein a live-attenuated CHIKV genome is delivered using the plasmid DNA. Immunization DNA plasmid was highly efficient and produced nAbs in 100% of the mice that were immunized. No viremia was detected in any animal post-challenge just like the deletion DNA vaccines. This candidate has a very low reversion frequency for the mutations (Hidajat et al., 2016). Thus, the DNA-based infectious-particle vaccines are speculated to be safer than live attenuated ones while simultaneously preserving the positive characters of a live product.

Delivery of genomic sequences that encode for anti-CHIKV mAbs through a plasmid vector is another innovative DNA vaccine strategy that is being considered (Muthumani et al., 2016). Since the plasmids will be generating a biologically active antibody, an immediate immune response will be generated along with the production of therapeutic antibodies. Such DNA vaccines will not have a long incubation phase as compared to traditional antigen-generating vaccines.

DNA vaccines offer several advantages like the ease of production and safety. DNA is a relatively stable molecule and has a long shelf life as it is much more durable in cold-chain storage conditions. The ability of DNA vaccines to developing both cell-mediated and humoral immunity is substantial and is found to be particularly helpful for the pathogens for which we do not know whether the protection is imparted by cell-mediated or by humoral immunity. However, the low immunogenicity of the vaccine in humans requires larger doses and repeated boosters (Ferraro et al., 2011). DNA uptake and use of adjuvants are some of the challenges posed by this approach (Sällberg et al., 2015).

Protein Subunit Vaccines

Using CHIKV-specific proteins that could elicit protective immunity, for subunit vaccines provides numerous advantages that include safety and scalability. Since there is no viral genome or infectious particle they are much safer than live viruses. The individual proteins can also be easily produced in large-scale manufacturing facilities. Since the immunogenicity of the CHIKV E1 and E2 and their role in generating protective immunity is well understood, this has led to the formulation of subunit vaccines based on these glycoproteins. One of the potential subunit vaccines against CHIKV has been synthesized using a baculovirus expression system. This particular vaccine utilizes recombinant E1 and E2 proteins along with the associated peptides of E3 and 6K/TF (Metz et al., 2011). The development of these proteins in insect systems lead to questions about their appropriate cleavage and glycosylation; however, in the Western blot analyses, it was seen that both the proteins had the expected molecular weights, were N-glycosylated, at least partially, and were secreted (Metz et al., 2011). Subunit vaccines generated neutralizing antibodies against the E2 recombinant protein. They also induced nAbs in mice (AG129) but at levels lower than intact VLPs (Metz et al., 2013).

Some other subunit vaccine candidates are based on the E1 or E2 protein of CHIKV but without E3 or 6K/TF associated peptides and have been produced using bacterial expression systems (Kumar et al., 2012; Khan et al,. 2012). The E2 protein along with a suitable adjuvant mounts a strong immune response and generates high nAb titers in mouse models. Immunization of BALB/c mice with the truncated E2 protein also exhibited complete protection against the disease by mounting a cell-mediated immune response (Kumar et al., 2012).

Live Attenuated Vaccines

Live attenuated vaccines are typically produced by the repeated passage of the infectious pathogen in the cell culture. However, advancements in alphavirus reverse genetic technology and systems have allowed for the synthesis of rationally designed, attenuated vaccines, which consist of very specific mutations or changes in their genome which improves the vaccine's specificity, safety profile, and expression. Expression at high levels offers protection with just a single dose. Despite all these advantages, there are chances of reversions that make the live attenuated vaccines disadvantageous.

One of the most developed live attenuated vaccine candidates for CHIKV is a full-length CHIKV clone derived from a wild-type ECSA strain, in which the natural subgenomic promoter has been replaced with the IRES (internal ribosome entry site) of an encephalomyocarditis virus (Plante et al., 2011). Host range gets functionally altered by the IRES element, as viruses derived from the cDNA are unable to replicate in mosquitoes. Thus, even if a vaccinee developed viremia after immunization, it won't get transmitted to mosquitoes, hence making it a safer vaccine. The same approach has been used for the synthesis of VEEV chimeric viruses. The engineered viruses express structural polyprotein in abundance and pose no risk of reversion to the wild type (Guerbois et al., 2013). Furthermore, since the nonstructural CHIKV elements are included accentuating specific immune response and diminishing the degree of attenuation that typically accompanies chimeric alphaviruses, especially the ones that are created on an already attenuated parent strain.

CHIKV-IRES vaccine showed satisfactory results in mouse models. No virus could be detected in any of the tissue samples (Plante et al., 2011). When the immunized mice were challenged with a wild-type CHIKV strain, no signs of illness were reported (Plante et al., 2011).

Additionally, by mutating specific virus sequences that are associated with special functions, CHIKV can be attenuated to make a potent vaccine. One novel strategy has been to modify the nucleolar localization sequence (NoLS) present in the N terminal region of the capsid protein. This alteration in the gene sequence prevents translocation of the capsid protein into the host cell nucleolus. Such a mutation leads to the cessation of host cell transcription in encephalitic alphaviruses, however, the effect on arthralgic alphaviruses is still not known.

Taylor and co-workers mutated this site in the virus (CHIKV-NoLS) and observed a reduction in replication of CHIKV, both in mosquito and mammalian cells. Mice (C57BL/6) infected with the mutant did not display any signs of the disease. The immunized mice also exhibited immunity against the Ross River virus (RRV) (Taylor et al., 2017).

Recombinant Vector Vaccine

The MV-CHIK is a recombinant measles virus-based vaccine expressing the envelop glycoproteins of the ECSA strain of CHIKV. The preclinical studies presented satisfactory results. On a lethal CHIKV challenge, the immunized mice mounted an effective immune response and showed protection against the disease.

In phase 1 clinical trials, after administration of the first dose, MV-CHIK elicited a strong nAb response in all of the immunized subjects. No occurrences of adverse events were reported. This immune response was further boosted after administration of the second dose. No significant immunogenic response was mounted against the vaccine vector (Tharmarajah et al., 2017). From the Phase 2 trials, it was reported that MV-CHIK has excellent safety and tolerability and offers good immunogenicity. Thus, MV-CHIK is a promising vaccine candidate for CHIKF prevention (Reisinger et al., 2019).

Conclusion

The rampant rise of CHIKV around the world has created an urgency for therapeutics and prophylactics. So far vaccines have been mankind's best option to combat any disease particularly those caused by viruses. Successful large-scale immunization campaigns have helped in the eradication of smallpox and control of deadly pathogens like polio, rabies, measles, mumps, rubella, etc. The long-term protection imparted by vaccines makes it the most effective method to prevent any disease.

However, developing vaccines is a tedious task. The requisite for an extremely high safety profile makes it difficult for them to surpass the series of stringent tests and trials. Thus out of many, only a few vaccine candidates rarely get approved. Furthermore, large-scale production of vaccines requires adequate infrastructure and sufficient amounts of capital. Because of this, impoverished countries that are already suffering from a scarcity of resources may become heavily dependent on imports due to their limited production capacity. As seen in the current scenario of the COVID-19 pandemic, a precise and meticulous strategy must be employed to ensure the equitable distribution of vaccines. Strategies to prevent hoarding of the world's vaccine supply must be devised. To ensure that such instances are not repeated one must consider waiving patent rights so that other manufacturers can also produce vaccines. Additionally, some vaccines may require booster doses which may discourage their widespread use among the population.

On the other hand, passive immunization by mAbs/nAbs does prove to be highly efficacious due to the wide array of effector mechanisms they employ. Monoclonal Abs specific to different targets can be administered in the form of a cocktail as a probable remedy for CHIKV. But due to their potential risk of hypersensitivity, immunosuppression, and high manufacturing cost, Abs-based therapies are not preferred. There is so much that is still unknown about CHIKV. The global research community needs to come together to find answers to these questions.

REFERENCES

Akahata, Wataru, Zhi-Yong Yang, Hanne Andersen, Siyang Sun, Heather A. Holdaway, Wing-Pui Kong, Mark G. Lewis, et al. 2010. "A Virus-like Particle Vaccine for Epidemic Chikungunya Virus Protects Nonhuman Primates against Infection." *Nature Medicine* 16 (3): 334–38. https://doi.org/10.1038/nm.2105.

Bao, Huihui, Aarti A. Ramanathan, Omkar Kawalakar, Senthil G. Sundaram, Colleen Tingey, Charoran B. Bian, Nagarajan

Muruganandam, et al. 2013. "Nonstructural Protein 2 (nsP2) of Chikungunya Virus (CHIKV) Enhances Protective Immunity Mediated by a CHIKV Envelope Protein Expressing DNA Vaccine." *Viral Immunology* 26 (1): 75–83. https://doi.org/10.1089/vim.2012.0061.

Bournazos, Stylianos, and Jeffrey V. Ravetch. 2015. "Fcγ Receptor Pathways during Active and Passive Immunization." *Immunological Reviews* 268 (1): 88–103.

Bournazos, Stylianos, David J. DiLillo, and Jeffrey V. Ravetch. 2015. "The Role of Fc-FcγR Interactions in IgG-Mediated Microbial Neutralization." *The Journal of Experimental Medicine* 212 (9): 1361–69.

Bruhns, Pierre. 2012. "Properties of Mouse and Human IgG Receptors and Their Contribution to Disease Models." *Blood* 119 (24): 5640–49.

Casadevall, Arturo, and Liise-Anne Pirofski. 2020. "The Convalescent Sera Option for Containing COVID-19." *The Journal of Clinical Investigation* 130 (4): 1545–48. https://doi.org/10.1172/JCI138003.

Chang, Lee-Jah, Kimberly A. Dowd, Floreliz H. Mendoza, Jamie G. Saunders, Sandra Sitar, Sarah H. Plummer, Galina Yamshchikov, et al. 2014. "Safety and Tolerability of Chikungunya Virus-like Particle Vaccine in Healthy Adults: A Phase 1 Dose-Escalation Trial." *The Lancet* 384 (9959): 2046–52. https://doi.org/10.1016/S0140-6736(14)61185-5.

Chen, Grace L., Emily E. Coates, Sarah H. Plummer, Cristina A. Carter, Nina Berkowitz, Michelle Conan-Cibotti, Josephine H. Cox, et al. 2020. "Effect of a Chikungunya Virus-Like Particle Vaccine on Safety and Tolerability Outcomes: A Randomized Clinical Trial." *JAMA: The Journal of the American Medical Association* 323 (14): 1369–77. doi:10.1001/jama.2020.2477.

Clinical Trial for Safety and Immunogenicity of a Chikungunya Vaccine, VRC-CHKVLP059-00-VP, in Healthy Adults: Accessed in April 2021 https://clinicaltrials.gov/ct2/show/results/NCT02562482.

Couderc, Thérèse, Nassirah Khandoudi, Marc Grandadam, François Prost, and Marc Lecuit Catherine Visse, Nicolas Gangneux, Sébastian Bagot, Jean "Prophylaxis and Therapy for Chikungunya Virus Infection." *The*

Journal of Infectious disease 200, no. 4 (2009): 516-23. Accessed May 3, 2021. http://www.jstor.org/stable/40255029.

Erasmus, Jesse H., Shannan L. Rossi, and Scott C. Weaver. 2016. "Development of Vaccines for Chikungunya Fever." *The Journal of Infectious Diseases* 214 (suppl 5): S488–96. https://doi.org/10.1093/infdis/jiw271.

Ferraro, Bernadette, Matthew P. Morrow, Natalie A. Hutnick, Thomas H. Shin, Colleen E. Lucke, and David B. Weiner. 2011. "Clinical Applications of DNA Vaccines: Current Progress." *Clinical Infectious Diseases: An Official Publication of the Infectious Diseases Society of America* 53 (3): 296–302. https://doi.org/10.1093/cid/cir334.

Fox, Julie M., Vicky Roy, Bronwyn M. Gunn, Ling Huang, Melissa A. Edeling, Matthias Mack, Daved H. Fremont, et al. 2019. "Optimal Therapeutic Activity of Monoclonal Antibodies against Chikungunya Virus Requires Fc-FcγR Interaction on Monocytes." *Science Immunology*. https://doi.org/10.1126/sciimmunol.aav5062.

Freitas, André Ricardo Ribas, Maria Rita Donalisio, and Pedro María Alarcón-Elbal. 2018. "Excess Mortality and Causes Associated with Chikungunya, Puerto Rico, 2014-2015." *Emerging Infectious Diseases* 24 (12): 2352–55. https://doi.org/10.3201/eid2412.170639.

Getahun, Andrew, and John C. Cambier. 2015. "Of ITIMs, ITAMs, and ITAMis: Revisiting Immunoglobulin Fc Receptor Signaling." *Immunological Reviews*. https://doi.org/10.1111/imr.12336.

Goodridge, Helen S., David M. Underhill, and Nicolas Touret. 2012. "Mechanisms of Fc Receptor and Dectin-1 Activation for Phagocytosis." *Traffic* 13 (8): 1062–71.

Goo, Leslie, Kimberly A. Dowd, Tsai-Yu Lin, John R. Mascola, Barney S. Graham, Julie E. Ledgerwood, and Theodore C. Pierson. 2016. "A Virus-Like Particle Vaccine Elicits Broad Neutralizing Antibody Responses in Humans to All Chikungunya Virus Genotypes." *The Journal of Infectious Diseases* 214 (10): 1487–91. https://doi.org/10.1093/infdis/jiw431.

Guerbois, Mathilde, Eugenia Volkova, Naomi L. Forrester, Shannan L. Rossi, Ilya Frolov, and Scott C. Weaver. 2013. "IRES-Driven

Expression of the Capsid Protein of the Venezuelan Equine Encephalitis Virus TC-83 Vaccine Strain Increases Its Attenuation and Safety." *PLoS Neglected Tropical Diseases* 7 (5): e2197. https://doi.org/10.1371/journal.pntd.0002197.

Hallengärd, David, Maria Kakoulidou, Aleksei Lulla, Beate M. Kümmerer, Daniel X. Johansson, Margit Mutso, Valeria Lulla, et al. 2014. "Novel Attenuated Chikungunya Vaccine Candidates Elicit Protective Immunity in C57BL/6 Mice." *Journal of Virology* 88 (5): 2858–66. https://doi.org/10.1128/JVI.03453-13.

Hey, Adam. 2015. "History and Practice: Antibodies in Infectious Diseases." *Microbiology Spectrum* 3 (2): AID – 0026–2014. https://doi.org/10.1128/microbiolspec.AID-0026-2014.

Hidajat, Rachmat, Brian Nickols, Naomi Forrester, Irina Tretyakova, Scott Weaver, and Peter Pushko. 2016. "Next Generation Sequencing of DNA-Launched Chikungunya Vaccine Virus." *Virology* 490 (March): 83–90. https://doi.org/10.1016/j.virol.2016.01.009.

Hucke, Friederike I, Joachim J Bugert. 2020. "Current and Promising Antivirals Against Chikungunya Virus." *Front Public Health*. 2020 Dec 15;8:618624. doi: 10.3389/fpubh.2020.618624. PMID: 33384981; PMCID: PMC7769948.

Jin, J., & Simmons, G. (2019). Antiviral Functions of Monoclonal Antibodies against Chikungunya Virus. *Viruses*, *11*(4), 305. https://doi.org/10.3390/v11040305.

Jin, Jing, Jesús G. Galaz-Montoya, Michael B. Sherman, Stella Y. Sun, Cynthia S. Goldsmith, Eileen T. O'Toole, Larry Ackerman, et al. 2018. "Neutralizing Antibodies Inhibit Chikungunya Virus Budding at the Plasma Membrane." *Cell Host & Microbe*. https://doi.org/10.1016/j.chom.2018.07.018.

Jin, Jing, Nathan M. Liss, Dong-Hua Chen, Maofu Liao, Julie M. Fox, Raeann M. Shimak, Rachel H. Fong, et al. 2015. "Neutralizing Monoclonal Antibodies Block Chikungunya Virus Entry and Release by Targeting an Epitope Critical to Viral Pathogenesis." *Cell Reports* 13 (11): 2553–64.

Kam, Yiu-Wing, Fok-Moon Lum, Teck-Hui Teo, Wendy W. L. Lee, Diane Simarmata, Sumitro Harjanto, Chong-Long Chua, et al. 2012. "Early Neutralizing IgG Response to Chikungunya Virus in Infected Patients Targets a Dominant Linear Epitope on the E2 Glycoprotein." *EMBO Molecular Medicine* 4 (4): 330–43. https://doi.org/10.1002/emmm.201200213.

Kaur, Simran Preet, and Vandana Gupta. 2020. "COVID-19 Vaccine: A Comprehensive Status Report." *Virus Research* 288 (October): 198114.

Khan, Mohsin, Rekha Dhanwani, Putcha Venkata Lakshamana Rao, and Manmohan Parida. 2012. "Subunit Vaccine Formulations Based on Recombinant Envelope Proteins of Chikungunya Virus Elicit Balanced Th1/Th2 Response and Virus-Neutralizing Antibodies in Mice." *Virus Research* 167 (2): 236–46. https://doi.org/10.1016/j.virusres.2012.05.004.

Kindt, Thomas J., Richard A. Goldsby, Barbara A. Osborne, and Janis Kuby. 2007. *Kuby Immunology*. Macmillan.

Kumar, Manish, A. B. Sudeep, and Vidya A. Arankalle. 2012. "Evaluation of Recombinant E2 Protein-Based and Whole-Virus Inactivated Candidate Vaccines against Chikungunya Virus." *Vaccine* 30 (43): 6142–49. https://doi.org/10.1016/j.vaccine.2012.07.072.

Lam, Shirley, Min Nyo, Patchara Phuektes, Chow Wenn Yew, Yee Joo Tan, and Justin Jang Hann Chu. 2015. "A Potent Neutralizing IgM mAb Targeting the N218 Epitope on E2 Protein Protects against Chikungunya Virus Pathogenesis." *mAbs* 7 (6): 1178–94.

Leen Delang, Nidya Segura Guerrero, Ali Tas, Gilles Quérat, Boris Pastorino, Mathy Froeyen Kai Dallmeier, Dirk Jochmans, Piet Herdewijn, Felio Bello 6, Eric J Snijder, Xavier de Lamballerie, Byron Martina, Johan Neyts, Martijn J van Hemert, Pieter Leyssen 2014. "Mutations in the Chikungunya Virus Non-Structural Proteins Cause Resistance to Favipiravir (T-705), a Broad-Spectrum Antiviral." *The Journal of Antimicrobial Chemotherapy* 69 (10). https://doi.org/10.1093/jac/dku209.

Long, Feng, Rachel H. Fong, Stephen K. Austin, Zhenguo Chen, Thomas Klose, Andrei Fokine, Yue Liu, et al. 2015. "Cryo-EM Structures

Elucidate Neutralizing Mechanisms of Anti-Chikungunya Human Monoclonal Antibodies with Therapeutic Activity." *Proceedings of the National Academy of Sciences of the United States of America* 112 (45): 13898–903.

Lu, Jinghua, Jonathan Chu, Zhongcheng Zou, Nels B. Hamacher, Mark W. Rixon, and Peter D. Sun. 2015. "Structure of FcγRI in Complex with Fc Reveals the Importance of Glycan Recognition for High-Affinity IgG Binding." *Proceedings of the National Academy of Sciences of the United States of America* 112 (3): 833–38.

Mallilankaraman, Karthik, Devon J. Shedlock, Huihui Bao, Omkar U. Kawalekar, Paolo Fagone, Aarthi A. Ramanathan, Bernadette Ferraro, et al. 2011. "A DNA Vaccine against Chikungunya Virus Is Protective in Mice and Induces Neutralizing Antibodies in Mice and Nonhuman Primates." *PLoS Neglected Tropical Diseases* 5 (1): e928. https://doi.org/10.1371/journal.pntd.0000928.

Mavalankar, Dileep, Priya Shastri, Tathagata Bandyopadhyay, Jeram Parmar, and Karaikurichi V. Ramani. 2008. "Increased Mortality Rate Associated with Chikungunya Epidemic, Ahmedabad, India." *Emerging Infectious Diseases* 14 (3): 412–15. https://doi.org/10.3201/eid1403.070720.

Masrinoul, Promsin, Orapim Puiprom, Atsushi Tanaka, Miwa Kuwahara, Panjaporn Chaichana, Kazuyoshi Ikuta, Pongrama Ramasoota, and Tamaki Okabayashi. 2014. "Monoclonal Antibody Targeting Chikungunya Virus Envelope 1 Protein Inhibits Virus Release." *Virology* 464-465 (September): 111–17.

Metz, Stefan W., Corinne Geertsema, Byron E. Martina, Paulina Andrade, Jacco G. Heldens, Monique M. van Oers, Rob W. Goldbach, Just M. Vlak, and Gorben P. Pijlman. 2011. "Functional Processing and Secretion of Chikungunya Virus E1 and E2 Glycoproteins in Insect Cells." *Virology Journal* 8 (July): 353. https://doi.org/10.1186/1743-422X-8-353.

Metz, Stefan W., Byron E. Martina, Petra van den Doel, Corinne Geertsema, Albert D. Osterhaus, Just M. Vlak, and Gorben P. Pijlman. 2013. "Chikungunya Virus-like Particles Are More Immunogenic in a Lethal

AG129 Mouse Model Compared to Glycoprotein E1 or E2 Subunits." *Vaccine*. https://doi.org/10.1016/j.vaccine.2013.09.045.

Muthumani, Karuppiah, Peter Block, Seleeke Flingai, Nagarajan Muruganantham, Itta Krishna Chaaithanya, Colleen Tingey, Megan Wise,2016. "Rapid and Long-Term Immunity Elicited by DNA-Encoded Antibody Prophylaxis and DNA Vaccination Against Chikungunya Virus." *The Journal of Infectious Diseases* 214 (3): 369–78. https://doi.org/10.1093/infdis/jiw111.

Muthumani, Karuppiah, Katthikbabu M. Lankaraman, Dominick J. Laddy, Senthil G. Sundaram, Christopher W. Chung, Eric Sako, Ling Wu, et al. 2008. "Immunogenicity of Novel Consensus-Based DNA Vaccines against Chikungunya Virus." *Vaccine* 26 (40): 5128–34. https://doi.org/10.1016/j.vaccine.2008.03.060.

Nimmerjahn, Falk, and Jeffrey V. Ravetch. 2008. "Analyzing Antibody-Fc-Receptor Interactions." *Methods in Molecular Biology* 415: 151–62.

Pal, Pankaj, Julie M Fox, David W Hawman, Yan-Jang S Huang, Ilhem Messaoudi, Craig Kreklywich, Michae Denton, Alfred W Legasse, Patricia P Smith, Syd Johnson, Michael K Axthelm, Dana L Vanlandingham, Daniel N Streblow, Stephen Higgs, Thomas E Morrison, Michael S Diamond. 2014. "Chikungunya Viruses That Escape Monoclonal Antibody Therapy Are Clinically Attenuated, Stable, and Not Purified in Mosquitoes." *Journal of Virology*. https://doi.org/10.1128/jvi.01032-14.

Pal, Pankaj, Kimberly A. Dowd, James D. Brien, Melissa A. Edeling, Sergey Gorlatov, Syd Johnson, Iris Lee, et al. 2013. "Development of a Highly Protective Combination Monoclonal Antibody Therapy against Chikungunya Virus." *PLoS Pathogens* 9 (4): e1003312.

Pérez-Pérez, María-Jesús, Leen Delang, Lisa F. P. Ng, and Eva-María Priego. 2019. "Chikungunya Virus Drug Discovery: Still a Long Way to Go?" *Expert Opinion on Drug Discovery*. https://doi.org/10.1080/17460441.2019.1629413.

Plante, Kenneth, Eryu Wang, Charalambos D. Partidos, James Weger, Rodion Gorchakov, Konstantin Tsetsarkin, Erin M. Borland, et al. 2011. "Novel Chikungunya Vaccine Candidate with an IRES-Based

Attenuation and Host Range Alteration Mechanism." *PLoS Pathogens* 7 (7): e1002142. https://doi.org/10.1371/journal.ppat.1002142

Pluschke, Gerd, Gerard Bordmann, Maria E. Daoudaki, John D. Lambris, Mark Achtman, and Michael Neibert. 1989. "Isolation of Rat IgM to IgG Hybridoma Isotype Switch Variants and Analysis of the Efficiency of Rat Ig in Complement Activation." *European Journal of Immunology* 19 (1): 131–35. https://doi.org/10.1002/eji.1830190121.

Porta, Jason, Joyce Jose, John T. Roehrig, Carol D. Blair, Richard J. Kuhn, and Michael G. Rossmann. 2014. "Locking and Blocking the Viral Landscape of an Alphavirus with Neutralizing Antibodies." *Journal of Virology* 88 (17): 9616–23. https://doi.org/10.1128/jvi.01286-14.

Powers, Ann M., Aaron C. Brault, Robert B. Tesh, and Scott C. Weaver. 2000. "Re-Emergence of Chikungunya and O'nyong-Nyong Viruses: Evidence for Distinct Geographical Lineages and Distant Evolutionary Relationships." *Microbiology*. https://doi.org/10.1099/0022-1317-81-2-471.

Radaev, S., S. Motyka, W. H. Fridman, C. Sautes-Fridman, and P. D. Sun. 2001. "The Structure of a Human Type III Fcgamma Receptor in Complex with Fc." *The Journal of Biological Chemistry* 276 (19): 16469–77.

Reisinger, Emil C., Roland Tschismarov, Eckhard Beubler, Ursula Wiedermann, Christa Firbas, Micha Loebermann, Andrea Pfeiffer, Matthias Muellner, Erich Tauber, and Katrin Ramsauer. 2019. "Immunogenicity, Safety, and Tolerability of the Measles-Vectored Chikungunya Virus Vaccine MV-CHIK: A Double-Blind, Randomised, Placebo-Controlled and Active-Controlled Phase 2 Trial." *The Lancet* 392 (10165): 2718–27. https://doi.org/10.1016/S0140-6736(18)32488-7.

Roques, Pierre, Karl Ljungberg, Beate M. Kümmerer, Leslie Gosse, Nathalie Dereuddre-Bosquet, Nicolas Tchitchek, David Hallengärd, et al. 2017. "Attenuated and Vectored Vaccines Protect Nonhuman Primates against Chikungunya Virus." *JCI Insight* 2 (6): e83527. https://doi.org/10.1172/jci.insight.83527.

Rupp, Jonathan C., Kevin J. Sokoloski, Natasha N. Gebhart, and Richard W. Hardy. 2015. "Alphavirus RNA Synthesis and Non-Structural Protein Functions." *Journal of General Virology.* https://doi.org/10.1099/jgv.0.000249.

Sällberg, Matti, Lars Frelin, Gustaf Ahlén, and Margaret Sällberg-Chen. 2015. "Electroporation for Therapeutic DNA Vaccination in Patients." *Medical Microbiology and Immunology* 204 (1): 131–35.

Schwartz, Olivier, and Matthew L. Albert. 2010. "Biology and Pathogenesis of Chikungunya Virus." *Nature Reviews Microbiology*. https://doi.org/10.1038/nrmicro2368.

Silva L.A., and Dermody T.S. 2017. "Chikungunya virus: epidemiology, replication, disease mechanisms, and prospective intervention strategies." *J Clin Invest.* Mar 1;127(3):737-749. doi: 10.1172/JCI84417. Epub 2017 Mar 1. PMID: 28248203; PMCID: PMC5330729.

Singh A. and Gupta V. 2021. SARS-CoV-2 therapeutics: how far do we stand from a remedy? *Pharmacol Rep.* 2021 Jan 3:1–19. doi: 10.1007/s43440-020-00204-0. Epub ahead of print. PMID: 33389724; PMCID: PMC7778692.

Smith, Scott A., Laurie A. Silva, Julie M. Fox, Andrew I. Flyak, Nurgun Kose, Gopal Sapparapu, Solomiia Khomandiak, et al. 2015. "Isolation and Characterization of Broad and Ultrapotent Human Monoclonal Antibodies with Therapeutic Activity against Chikungunya Virus." *Cell Host & Microbe* 18 (1): 86–95.

Sondermann, P., J. Kaiser, and U. Jacob. 2001. "Molecular Basis for Immune Complex Recognition: A Comparison of Fc-Receptor Structures." *Journal of Molecular Biology* 309 (3): 737–49.

Sparrow, Erin, Martin Friede, Mohamud Sheikh, and Siranda Torvaldsen. 2017. "Therapeutic Antibodies for Infectious Diseases." *Bulletin of the World Health Organization*. https://doi.org/10.2471/blt.16.178061.

Sun, Siyang, Ye Xiang, Wataru Akahata, Heather Holdaway, Pankaj Pal, Xinzheng Zhang, Michael S. Diamond, Gary J. Nabel, and Michael G. Rossmann. 2013. "Structural Analyses at Pseudo Atomic Resolution of Chikungunya Virus and Antibodies Show Mechanisms of Neutralization." *eLife* 2 (April): e00435.

Suhrbier A. 2019. "Rheumatic manifestations of chikungunya: emerging concepts and interventions." *Nat Rev Rheumatol.* Oct;15(10):597-611. doi: 10.1038/s41584-019-0276-9. Epub 2019 Sep 3. PMID: 31481759.

Taylor, Adam, Xiang Liu, Ali Zaid, Lucas Y. H. Goh, Jody Hobson-Peters, Roy A. Hall, Andres Merits, and Suresh Mahalingam. 2017. "Mutation of the N-Terminal Region of Chikungunya Virus Capsid Protein: Implications for Vaccine Design." *mBio*. https://doi.org/10.1128/mbio.01970-16.

Tharmarajah, Kothila, Suresh Mahalingam, and Ali Zaid. 2017. "Chikungunya: Vaccines and Therapeutics." *F1000Research*. https://doi.org/10.12688/f1000research.12461.1.

Tretyakova, Irina, Jason Hearn, Eryu Wang, Scott Weaver, and Peter Pushko. 2014. "DNA Vaccine Initiates Replication of Live Attenuated Chikungunya Virus *in Vitro* and Elicits Protective Immune Response in Mice." *The Journal of Infectious Diseases* 209 (12): 1882–90. https://doi.org/10.1093/infdis/jiu114

Wada, Yuji, Yasuko Orba, Michihito Sasaki, Shintaro Kobayashi, Michael J. Carr, Haruaki Nobori, Akihiko Sato, William W. Hall, and Hirofumi Sawa. 2017. "Discovery of a Novel Antiviral Agent Targeting the Nonstructural Protein 4 (nsP4) of Chikungunya Virus." *Virology* 505 (May): 102–12. https://doi.org/10.1016/j.virol.2017.02.014.

Weaver, Scott C., and Marc Lecuit. 2015. "Chikungunya Virus and the Global Spread of a Mosquito-Borne Disease." *New England Journal of Medicine*. https://doi.org/10.1056/nejmra1406035.

Weber, Christopher, Eva Berberich, Christine von Rhein, Lisa Henß, Eberhard Hildt, and Barbara S. Schnierle. 2017. "Identification of Functional Determinants in the Chikungunya Virus E2 Protein." *PLoS Neglected Tropical Diseases* 11 (1): e0005318. https://doi.org/10.1371/journal.pntd.0005318.

Zhang, Rong, Arthur S. Kim, Julie M. Fox, Sharmila Nair, Katherine Basore, William B. Klimstra, Rebecca Rimkunas, et al. 2018. "Mxra8 Is a Receptor for Multiple Arthritogenic Alphaviruses." *Nature* 557 (7706): 570–74.

In: Chikungunya
Editor: Phillip Galvan

ISBN: 978-1-53619-978-9

Chapter 4

RECENT ADVANCES IN CHIKUNGUNYA VIRUS THERAPEUTICS: AN OVERVIEW

Mohd Fardeen Husain Shahanshah[1], Himanshu Sehrawat[1], Chanuka Wijewardana[1], Sachin Pal[1], Amita Gupta[2], Prerna Diwan[1], Sanjay Gupta[3] and Vandana Gupta[1,*]

[1]Department of Microbiology, Ram Lal Anand College, University of Delhi, Benito Juarez Road, New Delhi, India
[2]Centre for Innovation in Infectious Disease Research, Education and Training, University of Delhi South Campus, Benito Juarez Marg, India
[3]Centre for Emerging Diseases, Department of Biotechnology, Jaypee Institute of Information Technology, Noida, India

ABSTRACT

Since its first presence in Tanzania in 1952, the Chikungunya virus (CHIKV) has caused several severe outbreaks and epidemics throughout

* Corresponding Author's E-mail: vandanagupta72@rediffmail.com, vandanagupta@rla.du.ac.in.

the world, affecting nearly 40 countries. This arthropod-borne virus is responsible for causing musculoskeletal inflammatory disease in humans. With rising global temperatures, that encourage the growth of the *Aedes* mosquito and lack of approved therapeutics, the risk of future outbreaks expanding beyond the confines of the tropics has significantly increased. As of now, there are no FDA-approved therapeutics available for the treatment of chikungunya however, many are in pipeline and are awaiting clinical trials. The recurring and sporadic CHIKV outbreaks and epidemics mandate the need for potent therapeutics against the virus. In this chapter, we intend to provide an overview of the potential therapeutics that have been proposed and developed for CHIKV.

Abbreviations

CHIKV:	Chikungunya virus
CHIKF:	Chikungunya fever
nsP:	nonstructural proteins
FDA:	Food and Drug Administration
IFN:	Interferon
NSAID:	Non-steroidal anti-inflammatory drugs

1. Introduction

Chikungunya virus (CHIKV), an alphavirus causes febrile musculoskeletal inflammatory disease in humans. Since its discovery in Tanzania in 1952, this arthropod-borne virus has prompted several outbreaks and epidemics across countries of Southeast Asia, South America, and Central Africa. However, with rising global temperatures encouraging the growth of its vector *Aedes aegypti* and *Aedes albopictus*, the incidence of this viral disease has increased significantly and has expanded to even temperate territories such as Northern Asia, Southern Europe, and the North America. (Schwartz and Albert 2010; Pérez-Pérez et al., 2019). The bite from an infected mosquito transmits this disease to humans and results in an illness that causes severe morbidity. The incubation period lasts for 2-4 days followed by an abrupt onset of clinical disease wherein the patient suffers from high fever, headache, rigors, petechial or maculopapular rash, and the hallmarks of the disease, myalgia, and polyarthralgia (Silva & Dermody 2017; Schwartz and Albert 2010; Weaver and Lecuit 2015). Polyarthralgia mainly affects the small joints of ankles, wrists, and phalanges, along with the larger joints such as the elbow and the knee. The muscle and joint pain can be incapacitating and may persist for months or even years (Suhrbier 2019). It is worth mentioning that CHIKF progresses without a prodromal phase and symptoms occur only when viremia has set in (Schwartz and Albert 2010). The acute CHIKF disease lasts for almost a week during which the rising viral titer triggers Type 1 (IFNs) interferon-mediated innate immune response (Schwartz and Albert 2010). Following the acute phase, the convalescent phase is characterized by clearance of viremia and alleviation of symptoms (Schwartz and Albert 2010). The illness can manifest into a chronic disease and induce long-term arthralgia. Studies from recent outbreaks have suggested that old patients are much more predisposed/susceptible to developing a chronic disease however, the exact cause and markers still haven't been identified and call for further research (Schwartz and Albert 2010). Neonates, patients who are aged and have existing comorbidities like diabetes, cardiovascular, respiratory, and neurological disorders are much more prone to developing a critical condition and succumbing to the infection. Even though the case fatality rate has been estimated to be 1 in 1000, the high degree of morbidity associated with Chikungunya is a source of grave concern (Schwartz and Albert 2010). Moreover, the scarcity of licensed therapeutics makes it burdensome and challenging to manage. To lessen the socio-economic losses experienced during a chikungunya outbreak and epidemic, there is an immediate need for the development of efficacious CHIKV antiviral therapeutics (Wada et al., 2017). Most current strategies are limited to managing the symptom using antipyretics, non-steroidal anti-inflammatory drugs (NSAIDs), and vector control with mosquito repellents and insecticides (Pérez-Pérez et al., 2019; Delang et al., 2014). The first step towards the development of effective antivirals would be reviewing the reported promising leads.

This chapter is a humble attempt to provide the reader with a comprehensive overview of the probable therapeutics including antiviral drugs and phytochemicals that have been proposed and are under development for the treatment of CHIKV.

1.1. Virology of CHIKV

CHIKV is an alphavirus that belongs to the family Togaviridae. This medium sized, enveloped virus particle has a diameter of 60-70 nm encasing 11.9 kb long, positive sense, single-stranded RNA genome which has a 7-methyl-GpppA cap at its 5' terminus and poly(A) tail at its 3' terminus (Rupp et al., 2015). The genome comprises of two open reading frames, ORF1 and ORF2, out of which the former encodes for the 4 non-structural proteins involved in the formation of the replicative enzyme complex and facilitate RNA synthesis while the latter encodes for the 5 structural proteins that are involved in the assembly of new virus particles (Pérez-Pérez et al., 2019).

Two-thirds of the 5' end of its genome translates into nonstructural polyprotein (nsP-1234) and the rest replicates into a subgenomic positive-strand mRNA referred to as 26S RNA, which ultimately translates into the five structural proteins (Khan et al., 2002; Solignat et al., 2009; Pérez-Pérez et al., 2019). The genome organisation and gene products have been illustrated in figure 1 (Kumar, Kumar, and Giri 2019; Rupp et al., 2015; Solignat et al., 2009; Kaur et al., 2020).

E1, E2, and E3 glycoproteins, 6k, and capsid protein (CP) are the five structural proteins of CHIKV. The genome is enclosed within the capsid protein which in turn is surrounded by a host-derived lipid envelope that is decorated with E1 and E2 spike glycoproteins (Rupp et al., 2015). The spike proteins mediate virus particle attachment and entry to the host cell (Pérez-Pérez et al., 2019; Solignat et al., 2009). The exact role of E3 glycoprotein is not yet known, however, observations suggest that it may have a crucial role in virus maturation (Pérez-Pérez et al., 2019; Solignat et al., 2009). Lastly, 6k protein serves as a virporin that creates cation-selective channels in the plasma membrane of the infected cells and facilitates the release of newly formed virus particles (Pérez-Pérez et al., 2019; Lombardi Pereira et al., 2019; Weaver and Lecuit, 2015).

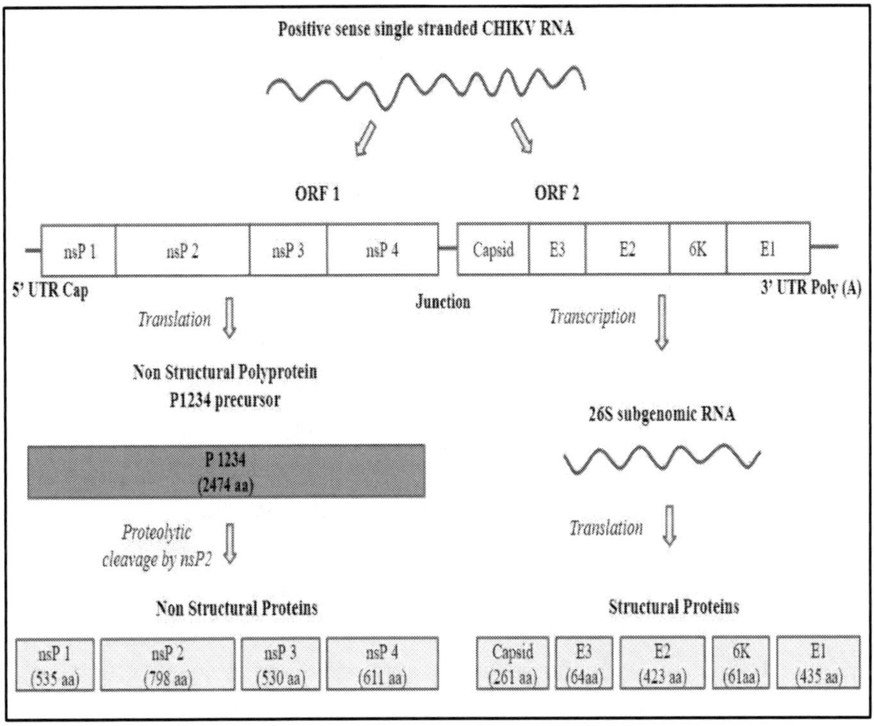

Figure 1. Genome Organisation and Gene Products (self-drawn).

The four nsPs of CHIKV namely, nsP1, nsP2, nsP3, and nsP4 together they play an essential role in viral replication and its regulation by forming the replicative enzyme complex. With its methyltransferase (MTase) and guanylyltransferase (GTase) activity, nsP1 prevents degradation of the newly synthesized viral RNA by adding a cap and a poly(A) tail to it. nsP2 is a multifunctional protein having both helicase and proteolytic activity. The processing of the P1234 polyprotein precursor is catalysed by this protein. Due to the indispensable function of nsP2, it is considered to be an attractive target for antivirals. On the contrary, nsP3 is a functionally ambiguous protein whose exact role is still unclear. It supposedly participates in the synthesis of both negative and positive-strand RNA molecules in conjunction with other nonstructural proteins. Finally, nsp4 is the RNA-dependent RNA polymerase that plays a central role in the replication process of the virus (Subudhi et al., 2018).

1.2. Pathogenesis of CHIKV

Following the bite of an infected *Aedes* mosquito, the virus enters the skin fibroblast and starts to replicate (Deeba et al., 2016). The E1, E2 spike glycoproteins present on the envelope of the virus aid in the attachment and aggregation of the virus particles onto the host cell (Schnierle 2019). The precise mechanism for entry of the virus into the target cell is still under contention, however, it has been suggested that CHIKV may resort to multiple pathways such as clathrin-mediated endocytosis, epidermal growth factor receptor substrate 15 (Eps15)-dependent pathway which is clathrin-independent and macropinocytosis to establish the infection (Schnierle 2019; Lombardi Pereira et al., 2019).

The acidic pH of the endocytic vesicles coated with clathrin enables uncoating of the virus in the target cell. On the contrary, macropinosomes are uncoated, large, actin-dependent vesicles involved in nonspecific uptake of extracellular components. Stimulation of the growth factor receptors by the virus initiates their formation and transduces a signal within the host cell that results in actin polarization and causes uptake of macropinosomes bound CHIKV (Schnierle 2019).

Once inside the host cell, the viral genomic RNA is translated by the host ribosomes into nonstructural polyprotein precursors (nsP1234). The polyprotein undergoes autocatalysis yielding nsP123 polyprotein and nsP4. The RNA polymerase activity of nsP4 helps in synthesizing the complementary negative strand of the viral genome whereas the nsP123 polyprotein undergoes further cleavage and is processed into mature nsP1, nsP2, and nsP3. Together, these nsPs form the replication enzyme complex and aid in transcription of a full-length positive-sense genomic, as well as 26S subgenomic viral RNA (Pérez-Pérez et al., 2019; Kaur et al., 2020). The subgenomic RNA gives rise to structural proteins. During the later stages of its replicative cycle, the CHIKV nucleocapsid core assembles within the cytoplasm. The assembled particle buds out through the plasma membrane and acquires a lipid envelope giving rise to a mature and infectious proge ny (Kaur et al., 2020; Pérez-Pérez et al., 2019; Solignat et al., 2009).

The virions released from the skin fibroblasts circulate to other parts of the body via blood and infect cells of the liver, muscle satellite, joint fibroblasts, synovial tissues, lymph nodes, and even the brain. This explains why people suffer from debilitating muscle and joint pain during CHIKV infections. Furthermore, in some cases, CHIKF has been found to be associated with neurological complications like encephalitis and encephalopathy, especially in case of vertical transmission of the virus, from infected mothers to the neonates (Weaver and Lecuit 2015; Schwartz and Albert 2010).

2. Therapeutics

A variety of therapeutics has been developed and proposed to work against CHIKV. The succeeding sections deals with a detailed discussion of these strategies.

2.1. Small Molecule Inhibitors (SMIs)

Small molecule inhibitors are one of the many approaches that can be used as a modality of treatment for Chikungunya Fever. They have a low molecular weight and can target various steps of the viral life cycle thereby arresting the replication process and preventing further spread of the infection. Based on the virology of CHIKV, several targets for SMIs have been identified that have been tabulated in Table 1 (Schnierle 2019; Haese, Powers, and Streblow 2020; Kovacikova and van Hemert 2020).

Table 1. Possible targets for small molecule inhibitors

S.no	Mode of Action	Target Site	Reference
1.	Inhibition of the viral entry into the host cell	The attachment of the viral particle to the host cell is achieved by binding of a viral glycoprotein E2 with a receptor protein present on the host cell. The cell adhesion molecule designated as Mxra8 acts as an entry mediator for the virus. The molecular inhibitors can either shut down the function of the glycoprotein or the receptor.	(Schnierle 2019; Haese, Powers, and Streblow 2020)
2.	Inhibiting the structural proteins	The outer envelope of the virus contains spike-like structures consisting of two glycoproteins, E1 and E2, and possesses a cytoplasmic tail which interacts with the capsid protein and facilitates assembly and budding of Chikungunya virus through the host cell plasma membrane.	(Haese, Powers, and Streblow 2020)
3.	Inhibiting the non-structural proteins and genome replication.	The nsPs of CHIKV together form a replicative complex and play an essential role in viral genome replication. Inhibition of these crucial segments of the viral proteins will cause disruptions in the viral replication and their functions.	(Kovacikova and van Hemert 2020; Haese, Powers, and Streblow 2020))
4.	Inhibiting host factors	Furin protease aids in the cleavage and activation of several viral glycoproteins. Enzymes like Dihydroorotate dehydrogenase (DHODH) and inosine monophosphate dehydrogenase are involved in nucleic acid base biosynthesis and hence can be targeted. Cellular kinases like Protein Kinase C (PKC) and Phosphatidylinositol 3-kinase (PI3K) may play an essential role in viral entry and hence these kinases along with their respective signaling pathways can be targeted. Protein disulfide isomerase (PDI) and Heat shock protein-90 (Hsp-90) are protein chaperones that are involved in CHIKV replication.	(Haese, Powers, and Streblow 2020)

SMIs will bind either to the target protein itself or to the receptor to carry out its inhibitory function (Haese, Powers, and Streblow 2020; Kovacikova and van Hemert 2020). In comparison to antibodies and proteins, the less complex nature of small molecule inhibitors makes them easier to manufacture synthetically thus reducing the cost of production. Furthermore, the analysis of such compounds and validation of their properties is fairly straightforward as problems of conformational differences or post-translational modification heterogeneity of proteins do not apply here (Alex Brown 2019)._An essential advantage of SMIs is that they can be administered orally and made into tablets, capsules, and even oral sprays as long as they have required properties (Alex brown 2019). SMIs can be further categorized into novel inhibitors or SMIs with no previous known use and repurposed drugs with a previously known medical use.

2.1.1. Novel Drugs

To date, none of the newly discovered and repurposed drugs against CHIKV have been licensed. Even though most of them do show inhibitory effects in in-vitro studies, but there still is a lack of knowledge about their mode of action and ADME properties. Since the breakthrough revelation of the crystal structures of several CHIKV proteins, the field of target-based drug designing and screening has grown significantly. Once the compound has been identified through screening, structural models are developed for further research and docking studies to gauge its activity and efficacy (Parashar and Cherian 2014).

In a study conducted by Lani and co-workers, the compounds Baicalein, Fisetin, and Quercetagetin exhibited inhibitory action on CHIKV infected Vero cells. These compounds had minimal cytotoxic activity. The phenotypic screening also revealed that Baicalein and Quercetagetin can act extracellularly on CHIKV (Lani et al., 2016). Table 2 enlists some of the anti-CHIKV novel drugs-like molecules.

Table 2. Novel Anti-CHIKV compounds

S.no	Novel Drug	EC50 value	Reference
1.	2-Oxo-4-(((4-oxo-3,4-dihydroquinazolin-2-yl)thio)methyl)-2H-chromen-7-yl Benzenesulfonate	19.1μM	(Hwu et al., 2015)
2.	2-Oxo-4-(((4-oxo-3,4-dihydroquinazolin-2-yl)thio)methyl)-2H-chromen-7-yl 4-Methylbenzenesulfonate	10.2μM	
3.	2-Oxo-4-(((4-oxo-3,4-dihydroquinazolin-2-yl)thio)methyl)-2H-chromen-7-yl 2-Nitrobenzenesulfonate	17.2μM	
4.	4-(((5-Methyl-6-oxo-1,6-dihydropyrimidin-2-yl)thio)methyl)-2-oxo-2H-chromen-7-yl 2-Nitrobenzenesulfonate	19.0μM	
5.	2-Oxo-4-(((6-oxo-1,6-dihydropyrimidin-2-yl)thio)methyl)-2H-chromen-7-yl Benzenesulfonate	13.0μM	
6.	MBZM-N-IBT (Hybrid of 2-methyl benzimidazole and isatin-β-thiosemicarbazone)	38.68μM	(Mishra et al., 2016)
7.	12-O-tetradecanoylphorbol 13-acetate	0.0003μM	(Bhakat and Soliman 2015)
8.	Trigowiin A	43.5μM	
9.	Prostratin	2.6μM	
10.	Phorbol	343μM	
11.	4α-12-O-tetradecanoylphorbol 13-acetate	2.8μM	
12.	3-(3′-acetylphenyl)-5-methyl-3H-(1,2,3)triazolo(4,5-d)pyrimidin-7(6H)-one (MADTP-314)	26 μM	(Delang et al., 2016)
13.	5-ethyl-3-(3-isopropoxyphenyl)-3H-(1,2,3)triazolo(4,5-d)-pyrimidin-7(6H)-one (MADTP-372	2.6 μM	

2.1.2 Repurposed Drugs

The Discovery of novel compounds is both time and resource-intensive. As a result, the unique approach of drug discovery known as drug repurposing or repositioning has been extensively explored to find new clinical use for existing approved drugs. Some known examples of drug repurposing include remdesivir, favipiravir, ivermectin, etc., for COVID-19, aspirin as a blood thinner, and many more. Since these drugs are pre-approved, their safety profiles have already been established and hence can directly enter the clinical trials (Pérez-Pérez et al., 2019).

Table 3. SMIs repositioned and proposed against CHIKV

Drug	Originally used for	Mode of Action	EC50 value	CC50 value	References
Ribavirin	Treatment of respiratory syncytial virus, human hepatitis C	Inhibits the polymerase enzyme (nsP4) of the virus and replication by inserting ribavirin triphosphate in the viral genome in place of GTP	5.5 μM	30.7 mM	(Subudhi et al., 2018; reviewed in Haese, Powers, and Streblow 2020; Pérez-Pérez et al., 2019; Franco et al., 2018; Ferreira et al., n.d.; Silva-Júnior et al., 2017; Ehteshami et al., 2017)
6-azauridine	Treatment of psoriasis	Inhibit viral genome replication	0.82 μM	51 μg/mL	(Pérez-Pérez et al., 2019; Franco et al., 2018; Ferreira et al., n.d.; Subudhi et al., 2018; Silva-Júnior et al., 2017; Ehteshami et al., 2017)
4-hydroxycytidine	Treatment of human hepatitis C	Inhibit viral replication by targeting viral polymerase, Increase the rate of mutagenesis	0.8 μM	7.7 μM (vero)	(Pérez-Pérez et al., 2019; Franco et al., 2018; Ferreira et al., n.d.; Subudhi et al., 2018; Silva-Júnior et al., 2017; Ehteshami et al., 2017)
Favipiravir	Treatment of influenza virus	Substitute for the RdRp (nsP4) of the virus and prevent the binding of ATP and GTP to the viral RdRp resulting in the inhibition of replication by inhibiting the enzyme RNA polymerase	20 μg/mL	-	(Subudhi et al. 2018; reviewed in Haese, Powers, and Streblow 2020)

Table 3. (Continued)

Drug	Originally used for	Mode of Action	EC50 value	CC50 value	References
Sofosbuvir	Treatment of human hepatitis C		2.7 µM	-	(Pérez-Pérez et al., 2019; Franco et al., 2018; Ferreira et al., n.d.; Subudhi et al., 2018; Silva-Júnior et al., 2017; Ehteshami et al., 2017)
Arbidol	Treatment of influenza	Inhibit the binding of the virus to host receptor and RNA replication of the virus	12 µM	376 µM	(Abdelnabi, Neyts, and Delang 2016; Delogu et al., 2011; reviewed in Haese, Powers, and Streblow 2020)
Chloro-quine	Treatment of malaria	By increasing the pH of the endosome, it inhibits the fusion of the virus to the endosomal membrane and stops the viral uncoating.	17.2µM	260 µM	(Khan et al., 2010; reviewed in Haese, Powers, and Streblow 2020)
Bafilomycin	Function as an ATPase inhibitor	Inhibit CHIKV entry to host	0.33 nM	0.003 µM	(Pérez-Pérez et al., 2019; Franco et al., 2018; Ferreira et al., n.d.; Subudhi et al., 2018; Silva-Júnior et al., 2017; Ehteshami et al., 2017)
Pimozide	Tourette's disorder	Disrupt various stages of the CHIKV lifecycle	0.28 µM	19.18 µM	(Pérez-Pérez et al., 2019; Franco et al., 2018; Ferreira et al., n.d.; Subudhi et al., 2018; Silva-Júnior et al., 2017; Ehteshami et al., 2017)

Drug	Originally used for	Mode of Action	EC50 value	CC50 value	References
5 – tetradecyloxy – 2 – furoic acid	Hyperlipidemias	Disrupt various stages of CHIKV lifecycle	0.15μM	60 μM	(Pérez-Pérez et al., 2019; Franco et al., 2018; Ferreira et al., n.d.; Subudhi et al., 2018; Silva-Júnior et al., 2017; Ehteshami et al., 2017)
Tivozanib	Renal cell cancer	Disrupt various stages of CHIKV lifecycle	0.8 μM	8.34 μM	(Pérez-Pérez et al., 2019; Franco et al., 2018; Ferreira et al., n.d.; Subudhi et al., 2018; Silva-Júnior et al., 2017; Ehteshami et al., 2017)
Mycophenolic acid	Function as an immunosuppressant to prevent organ transplant rejection.	Disrupt viral genome replication	0.1μM	30 μM	(Pérez-Pérez et al., 2019; Franco et al., 2018; Ferreira et al., n.d.; Subudhi et al., 2018; Silva-Júnior et al., 2017; Ehteshami et al., 2017)
Suramin	An antiparasitic used for the treatment of African sleeping sickness and river blindness.	Inhibits the entry of the virus in the host cell	80 μM	> 5 mM	(reviewed in Haese, Powers, and Streblow 2020)
Picolinic Acid	-	Inhibits the structural proteins responsible for capsid	-	-	(reviewed in Haese, Powers, and Streblow 2020)
Lobaric acid	-	Inhibits the functions of nsP1	9.9 μM	76.3 μM	(reviewed in Haese, Powers, and Streblow 2020)
Geldanamycin HS 10	Antineoplastic antibiotic	Inhibits the host protein chaperone HSP 90	-	-	(reviewed in Haese, Powers, and Streblow 2020)

Table 3 enlists selected SMIs which exhibited repurposing potential for the treatment of CHIKV.

2.2. Natural Inhibitors or Phytochemicals as Antivirals

From the earliest days of drug discovery, chemical compounds isolated from natural sources have been used as therapeutics for treating several ailments. Due to their minimal side effects and fewer chances of developing resistance, the potential of phytochemicals as antivirals has stimulated the interest of many. So far numerous phytochemicals have been proposed against CHIKV (Dias, Urban, and Roessner 2012; Bhakat and Soliman 2015).

Curcumin, an active compound present in turmeric was initially used to treat gastrointestinal diseases. Its potential as an antiviral was confirmed when curcumin-treated pseudotyped viral particles were unable to bind to the host cells and transmit from one cell to another. The compound was able to reduce the viral infection to a large extent but due to its sub-par solubility and bioavailability, the results obtained in in-vivo studies weren't that encouraging (Subudhi et.al 2018; Mounse et.al 2017; Bhakat and Soliman 2015).

A bioactive compound known as Silvestol extracted from the trees of *Aglaia* can selectively inhibit the eukaryotic initiation factor elf4A. Through its helicase activity, elf4A plays an important role during translation. Hence, silvestrol can stall the translation process and inhibit the synthesis of nsPs and structural proteins thereby limiting the infection of CHIKV (Henss et al., 2018). More studies are required to validate its efficacy.

Berberine is an alkaloid obtained from *the Berberis* plant that can obstruct CHIKV replication by minimizing the activity of mitogen-activated protein kinase signaling pathways (Bhakat and Soliman 2015). Another compound called Trigowiin A, a type of tigliane diterpenoid isolated from *Trigonostemon Hawaii*, a plant native to Vietnam has also been shown to possess inhibitory properties against CHIKV (Bhakat and Soliman 2015). Both these compounds can be optimized and made into potent antiviral drugs.

Epigallocatechin gallate (EGCG), a unique phytochemical commonly found in green tea is known for its antitumor, anti-inflammatory, antiviral, antibacterial, and anti-toxic properties. This compound hampers the entry of

CHIKV into the host cell when administered at a concentration of 10 micrograms per milliliter however it does not reduce viral infectivity due to its poor absorption and pharmacokinetics (Weber et al., 2015; Lee et al., 2002).

Table 4. Natural inhibitors proposed against CHIKV

S.no	Phytochemical	Isolated from	Activity
1.	Flavaglines	*Aglaia*	Inhibits the entry of viral particles into the host cells
2.	Lupenone	Madagascan plant	Target is unidentified
3.	Jatrophan esters	*Euphorbia spp.*	By using PKC mediated mechanism (yet to be verified)
4.	Silymarin	*Silybum Marianum*	Inhibition of post-entry stages of viral replication
5.	2-O-decanoylphorbol-13-acetate	*Croton mauritianus*	Inhibits CHIKV genome replication
6.	12-O-decanolyl -7-hydropero-xy-phorbol-5-ene-13-acetate	*Croton mauritianus*	Inhibits Chikungunya virus genome replication
7.	Trigowiin A	*Trigonostemo n hawaii*	Inhibition of the signal transduction enzyme protein kinase C
8.	Curcumin	Turmeric plant	Inhibits virus's ability to bind to the cells and its cell to cell transmission
9.	Silvestrol	*Aglaia spp.*	Inhibits the eukaryotic initiation factor elf4A thereby arresting the translation of viral nsP and structural proteins
10.	Berberine	*Berberis oblonga*	Inhibits mitogen-activated protein kinase signaling pathways
11.	Epigallocate-chin gallate	green tea	Inhibits the entry of viral particles into the host cells
12.	Harringtonine	*Cephalo-taxus Harringtonia*	Suppress the production of nsP3 and E2 proteins by inhibiting host protein translation machinery.

Harringtonine is a cephalotaxine alkaloid procured from *Cephalotaxus harringtonia*. This anti-CHIKV bioactive agent suppresses host protein translation machinery and inhibits the synthesis of viral nsP3 and E2 proteins. The viral replicative complex is rendered non-functional without nsP3 and hence halts the viral RNA replication (Kaur et al., 2013). The phytochemicals showing anti CHIKV activity have been summarised in the Table 4 as reviewed extensively by Bhakat and Soliman (2015); Hucke and Bugert (2020); Subudhi et al., (2018).

Conclusion

The damaging implications of CHIKV outbreaks and epidemics have been endured by nations all across the globe. Due to its persistent and erratic nature, a necessity for efficacious anti-CHIKV therapeutics has emerged. Owing to the existing knowledge gaps about the virus and its interaction with the host, the search for therapies has been long and strenuous. But with the collective efforts of scientists and clinicians, numerous antivirals against CHIKV have been proposed in the last few years. From the discovery of novel compounds to the repositioning of existing drugs, all approaches have given promising results in preclinical studies. However, most of the reported molecules fail to advance further and hence none of them have been approved for CHIKV treatment. Even after extensive studies in different cell culture systems and in-vivo infection models, the relative roles of CHIKV and the host immune system during acute and chronic infections are still unknown.

The ease with which small molecule inhibitors can be manufactured and administered makes them a favorable antiviral therapeutic candidate over monoclonal antibodies. However, because of their poor bioavailability and short life span, the risk of increased toxicity is high. In this regard, phytochemicals as antivirals can be preferable due to their negligible side effects. Although they do have poor pharmacokinetic properties and are difficult to synthesize/isolate. Novel drugs can be the next best alternative to all these therapies but the studies towards discovery of even one compound is highly time-consuming. Drug repositioning can help counter the aforementioned problem. However, the lack of literature on viral proteins makes the process of drug repositioning tedious and challenging.

With the successful development of mRNA-based vaccines, an avenue of opportunities has opened up. Alternative therapies based on RNA interference can be a potential game-changer. Small RNA transcripts that are complementary to specific gene targets can be designed to inhibit or regulate gene expression. Prospective target sites for these RNA antivirals can either be viral genes or the host accessory genes that facilitate viral entry/infection. Like any other therapy, RNAi-based antivirals have their own set of insufficiencies like drug delivery, bioavailability, specificity, and stability. Hence, further research is needed for its optimization.

Another modality of treatment that hasn't been explored enough is Interferon based therapy. Interferons are signaling molecules that play a pivotal role in suppressing viral infections during an innate immune response. If these endogenously produced proteins are administrated during viral infections, a heightened immune response can be generated and viral spread can be subdued. The efficacy of this treatment is still unknown and hence calls for additional studies.

The discovery of anti-CHIKV therapeutics is majorly dependent on research and filling the existing knowledge gaps. This can only be accelerated by pooling support from the scientific community and increasing the capital investment put into research.

References

Abdelnabi Rana, Johan Neyts, and Leen Delang. 2016. "Antiviral Strategies Against Chikungunya Virus." *Methods in Molecular Biology*. https://doi.org/10.1007/978-1-4939-3618-2_22.

Abraham Rachy, Debra Hauer, Robert Lyle McPherson, Age Utt, Ilsa T. Kirby, Michael S. Cohen, Andres Merits, Anthony K. L. Leung, and Diane E. Griffin. 2018. "ADP-Ribosyl-Binding and Hydrolase Activities of the Alphavirus nsP3 Macrodomain Are Critical for Initiation of Virus Replication." *Proceedings of the National Academy of Sciences of the United States of America* 115 (44): E10457–66. https://doi.org/10.1073/pnas.1812130115.

Aggarwal Megha, Rajesh Sharma, Pravindra Kumar, Manmohan Parida, and Shailly Tomar. 2015. "Kinetic Characterization of Trans-Proteolytic Activity of Chikungunya Virus Capsid Protease and Development of a FRET-Based HTS Assay." *Scientific Reports 5 (October): 14753.* https://doi.org/10.1038/srep14753.

Akhrymuk Ivan, Sergey V. Kulemzin, and Elena I. Frolova. 2012. "Evasion of the Innate Immune Response: The Old World Alphavirus nsP2 Protein Induces Rapid Degradation of Rpb1, a Catalytic Subunit of RNA Polymerase II." *Journal of Virology* 86 (13): 7180–91. https://doi.org/10.1128/JVI.00541-12.

Bassetto, Marcella, Tine De Burghgraeve, Leen Delang, Alberto Massarotti, Antonio Coluccia, Nicola Zonta, Valerio Gatti, et al., 2013. "Computer-Aided Identification, Design and Synthesis of a Novel Series of Compounds with Selective Antiviral Activity against Chikungunya Virus." *Antiviral Research* 98 (1): 12–18. https://doi.org/10.1021/acsomega.1c00625.

Brown, Alex, *A few Q and A about small molecule inhibitors* accessed on April 2021 https://www.pharmiweb.com/article/a-few-qas-about-small-molecule-inhibitors.

Cardona-Correa, Sara E., Lina María Castaño-Jaramillo, and Augusto Quevedo-Vélez. 2017. "(Vertical transmission of chikungunya virus infection. Case Report)." *Revista chilena de pediatria* 88 (2): 285–88. DOI: 10.4067/s0370-41062017000200015. [*Chilean Pediatrics Magazine*]

Caruthers, Jonathan M., and David B. McKay. 2002. "Helicase Structure and Mechanism." *Current Opinion in Structural Biology*. https://doi.org/10.1016/s0959-440x(02)00298-1.

Deeba, Farah, Asimul Islam, Syed Naqui Kazim, Irshad Hussain Naqvi, Shobha Broor, Anwar Ahmed, and Shama Parveen. 2016. "Chikungunya Virus: Recent Advances in Epidemiology, Host Pathogen Interaction and Vaccine Strategies." *Pathogens and Disease*. https://doi.org/10.1093/femspd/ftv119.

Delang 1, C Li, A Tas, G Quérat, I C Albulescu, T De Burghgraeve, N A Segura Guerrero 1, A Gigante,G Piorkowski, E Decroly, D Jochmans 1,

B Canard, EJ Snijder,MJ Pérez-Pérez, M J van Hemert, B Coutard, P Leyssen, J Neyts 2016. "The Viral Capping Enzyme nsP1: A Novel Target for the Inhibition of Chikungunya Virus Infection." *Scientific Reports* 6 (August): 31819. https://doi.org/ 10.1038/srep31819.

Delang, Leen, Nidya Segura Guerrero, Ali Tas, Gilles Quérat, Boris Pastorino, Mathy Froeyen Kai Dallmeier, Dirk Jochmans,Piet Herdewijn, Felio Bello 6, Eric J Snijder, Xavier de Lamballerie, Byron Martina, Johan Neyts, Martijn J van Hemert, Pieter Leyssen2014. "Mutations in the Chikungunya Virus Non-Structural Proteins Cause Resistance to Favipiravir (T-705), a Broad-Spectrum Antiviral." *The Journal of Antimicrobial Chemotherapy* 69 (10). https://doi.org/ 10.1093/jac/dku209.

Delogu, Ilenia, Boris Pastorino, Cécile Baronti, Antoine Nougairède, Emilie Bonnet, and Xavier de Lamballerie. 2011. "*In Vitro* Antiviral Activity of Arbidol against Chikungunya Virus and Characteristics of a Selected Resistant Mutant." *Antiviral Research*. https://doi.org/ 10.1016/ j.antiviral.2011.03.182.

Dias, Daniel A., Sylvia Urban, and Ute Roessner. 2012. "A Historical Overview of Natural Products in Drug Discovery." *Metabolites* 2 (2): 303–36.

Economopoulou, M Dominguez, B Helynck, D Sissoko, O Wichmann, P Quenel, P Germonneau, Quatresous (2009). Atypical Chikungunya virus infections: clinical manifestations, mortality and risk factors for severe disease during the 2005-2006 outbreak on Réunion. *Epidemiology and infection*, 137(4), 534–541. https://doi.org/ 10.1017/S0950268 808001167.

Ehteshami, Maryam, Sijia Tao, Keivan Zandi, Hui-Mien Hsiao, Yong Jiang, Emily Hammond, Franck Amblard, Olivia O. Russell, Andres Merits, and Raymond F. Schinazi. 2017. "Characterization of β-D-N4-Hydroxycytidine as a Novel Inhibitor of Chikungunya Virus." *Antimicrobial Agents and Chemotherapy*. https://doi.org/10.1128/ aac.02395-16.

Ferreira, André C., Patrícia A. Reis, Caroline S. de Freitas, Carolina Q. Sacramento, Lucas Villas Bôas Hoelz, Mônica M. Bastos, Mayara

Mattos, et al., n.d. *Beyond Members of the Flaviviridae Family, Sofosbuvir Also Inhibits Chikungunya Virus Replication.* https://doi.org/10.1101/360305.

Franco, Evelyn J., Jaime L. Rodriquez, Justin J. Pomeroy, Kaley C. Hanrahan, and Ashley N. Brown. 2018. "The Effectiveness of Antiviral Agents with Broad-Spectrum Activity against Chikungunya Virus Varies between Host Cell Lines." *Antiviral Chemistry & Chemotherapy* 26 (January): 2040206618807580. https://doi.org/ 10.1177/2040 206618807580.

Fros, Jelke J., Lee D. Major, Florine E. M. Scholte, Joy Gardner, Martijn J. van Hemert, Andreas Suhrbier, and Gorben P. Pijlman. 2015. "Chikungunya Virus Non-Structural Protein 2-Mediated Host Shut-off Disables the Unfolded Protein Response." *Journal of General Virology*. https://doi.org/10.1099/vir.0.071845-0.

Gasque, Philippe, Marie Christine Jaffar Bandjee, Marcela Mercado Reyes, and Diego Viasus. 2016. "Chikungunya Pathogenesis: From the Clinics to the Bench." *The Journal of Infectious Diseases* 214 (suppl 5): S446–48.

Gorbalenya, Alexander E. Eugene V. Koonin, 1993; Helicases: amino acid sequence comparisons and structure-function relationships, *Current Opinion in Structural Biology,* Volume 3, Issue https://doi.org/10.1016/ S0959-440X(05)80116-2.

Goyal, Manu, Anil Chauhan, Vishavdeep Goyal, Nishant Jaiswal, Shreya Singh, and Meenu Singh. 2018. "Recent Development in the Strategies Projected for Chikungunya Vaccine in Humans." *Drug Design, Development and Therapy* 12 (December): 4195–4206. https://doi.org/ 10.2147/DDDT.S181574.

Haese, Nicole, John Powers, and Daniel N. Streblow. 2020. "Small Molecule Inhibitors Targeting Chikungunya Virus." *Current Topics in Microbiology and Immunology*, January. https://doi.org/10.1007/ 82_2020_195.

Henss, Lisa, Tatjana Scholz, Arnold Grünweller, and Barbara S. Schnierle. 2018. "Silvestrol Inhibits Chikungunya Virus Replication." *Viruses* 10 (11). https://doi.org/10.3390/v10110592.

Hoarau, Jean-Jacques, Marie-Christine Jaffar Bandjee, Pascale Krejbich Trotot, Trina Das, Ghislaine Li-Pat-Yuen, Bérengère Dassa, Mélanie Denizot, et al., 2010. "Persistent Chronic Inflammation and Infection by Chikungunya Arthritogenic Alphavirus in Spite of a Robust Host Immune Response." *Journal of Immunology* 184 (10): 5914–27. https://doi.org/10.4049/jimmunol.0900255.

Hucke, Friederike I, Joachim J Bugert. 2020. "Current and Promising Antivirals Against Chikungunya Virus." *Front Public Health*. 2020 Dec 15;8:618624. doi: 10.3389/fpubh.2020.618624. PMID: 33384981; PMCID: PMC7769948.

Hwu, Jih Ru, Mohit Kapoor, Shwu-Chen Tsay, Chun-Cheng Lin, Kuo Chu Hwang, Jia-Cherng Horng, I-Chia Chen, Fa-Kuen Shieh, Pieter Leyssen, and Johan Neyts. 2015. "Benzouracil-Coumarin-Arene Conjugates as Inhibiting Agents for Chikungunya Virus." *Antiviral Research 118* (June): 103–9. https://doi.org/10.1016/j.antiviral. 2015.03.013.

Joyce, Jose, Jonathan E. Snyder, and Richard J. Kuhn. 2009. "A Structural and Functional Perspective of Alphavirus Replication and Assembly." *Future Microbiology* 4 (7): 837–56. https://doi.org/ 10.2217/fmb.09.59.

Karpe, Yogesh A., Pankaj P. Aher, and Kavita S. Lole. 2011. "NTPase and 5'-RNA Triphosphatase Activities of Chikungunya Virus nsP2 Protein." *PloS One* 6 (7): e22336. https://doi.org/10.1371/ journal.pone.0022336.

Kaur, Parveen, Laura Sandra Lello, Age Utt, Sujit Krishna Dutta, Andres Merits, and Justin Jang Hann Chu. 2020. "Bortezomib Inhibits Chikungunya Virus Replication by Interfering with Viral Protein Synthesis." *PLoS Neglected Tropical Diseases* 14 (5). https://doi. org/10.1371/journal.pntd.0008336.

Kaur, Parveen, Meerra Thiruchelvan, Regina Ching Hua Lee, Huixin Chen, Karen Caiyun Chen, Mah Lee Ng, and Justin Jang Hann Chu. 2013. "Inhibition of Chikungunya Virus Replication by Harringtonine, a Novel Antiviral That Suppresses Viral Protein Expression." *Antimicrobial Agents and Chemotherapy* 57 (1): 155–67. https://doi.org/10.1128/AAC.01467-12.

Khan, Afjal Hossain, Kouichi Morita, Maria Del Carmen Parquet, Futoshi Hasebe, Edward G. M. Mathenge, and Akira Igarashi. 2002. "Complete Nucleotide Sequence of Chikungunya Virus and Evidence for an Internal Polyadenylation Site." *The Journal of General Virology* 83 (Pt 12): 3075–84. https://doi.org/10.1099/0022-1317-83-12-3075.

Khan, Mohsin, S. R. Santhosh, Mugdha Tiwari, P. V. Lakshmana Rao, and Manmohan Parida. 2010. "Assessment of in Vitro Prophylactic and Therapeutic Efficacy of Chloroquine against Chikungunya Virus in Vero Cells." *Journal of Medical Virology* 82 (5): 817–24.

Kovacikova, Kristina, and Martijn J. van Hemert. 2020. "Small-Molecule Inhibitors of Chikungunya Virus: Mechanisms of Action and Antiviral Drug Resistance." *Antimicrobial Agents and Chemotherapy* 64 (12). https://doi.org/10.1128/AAC.01788-20.

Kumar, Prateek, Deepak Kumar, and Rajanish Giri. 2019. "Targeting the nsp2 Cysteine Protease of Chikungunya Virus Using FDA Approved Library and Selected Cysteine Protease Inhibitors." *Pathogens* 8 (3). https://doi.org/10.3390/pathogens8030128.

Lage, Olga Maria, María C. Ramos, Rita Calisto, Eduarda Almeida, Vitor Vasconcelos, and Francisca Vicente. 2018. "Current Screening Methodologies in Drug Discovery for Selected Human Diseases." *Marine Drugs* 16 (8). https://doi.org/10.3390/md16080279.

Lani, Rafidah, Pouya Hassandarvish, Meng-Hooi Shu, Wai Hong Phoon, Justin Jang Hann Chu, Stephen Higgs, Dana Vanlandingham, Sazaly Abu Bakar, and Keivan Zandi. 2016. "Antiviral Activity of Selected Flavonoids against Chikungunya Virus." *Antiviral Research* 133 (September): 50–61. https://doi.org/10.1016/j.antiviral.2016.07. 009.

Law, Yee-Song, Age Utt, Yaw Bia Tan, Jie Zheng, Sainan Wang, Ming Wei Chen, Patrick R. Griffin, Andres Merits, and Dahai Luo. 2019. "Structural Insights into RNA Recognition by the Chikungunya Virus nsP2 Helicase." *Proceedings of the National Academy of Sciences of the United States of America* 116 (19): 9558–67. https://doi. org/10.1073/pnas.1900656116.

Lee, Mao-Jung, Pius Maliakal, Laishun Chen, Xiaofeng Meng, Flordeliza Y. Bondoc, Saileta Prabhu, George Lambert, Sandra Mohr, and Chung

S. Yang. 2002. "Pharmacokinetics of Tea Catechins after Ingestion of Green Tea and (-)-Epigallocatechin-3-Gallate by Humans: Formation of Different Metabolites and Individual Variability." *Cancer Epidemiology, Biomarkers & Prevention: A Publication of the American Association for Cancer Research, Cosponsored by the American Society of Preventive Oncology* 11 (10 Pt 1): 1025–32.

Linder, P., P. F. Lasko, M. Ashburner, P. Leroy, P. J. Nielsen, K. Nishi, J. Schnier, and P. P. Slonimski. 1989. "Birth of the D-E-A-D Box." *Nature* 337 (6203): 121–22. https://doi.org/10.1038/337121a0.

Lombardi Pereira, Ana Paula, Helena Tiemi Suzukawa, Aline Miquelin do Nascimento, Aedra Carla Bufalo Kawassaki, Camila Regina Basso, Dayane Priscila Dos Santos, Kamila Falchetti Damasco, Laís Fernanda Machado, Marla Karine Amarante, and Maria Angelica Ehara Watanabe. 2019. "An Overview of the Immune Response and Arginase I on CHIKV Immunopathogenesis." *Microbial Pathogenesis* 135 (October): 103581. https://doi.org/10.1016/j.micpath.2019. 103581.

Lucas-Hourani, Marianne, Alexandru Lupan, Philippe Desprès, Sylviane Thoret, Olivier Pamlard, Joëlle Dubois, Catherine Guillou, Frédéric Tangy, Pierre-Olivier Vidalain, and Hélène Munier-Lehmann. 2013. "A Phenotypic Assay to Identify Chikungunya Virus Inhibitors Targeting the Nonstructural Protein nsP2." *Journal of Biomolecular Screening* 18 (2): 172–79. https://doi.org/10.1177/10870571124 60091.

Miner, Jonathan J., Lindsey E. Cook, Jun P. Hong, Amber M. Smith, Justin M. Richner, Raeann M. Shimak, Alissa R. Young, et al., 2017. "Therapy with CTLA4-Ig and an Antiviral Monoclonal Antibody Controls Chikungunya Virus Arthritis." *Science Translational Medicine.* https://doi.org/10.1126/scitranslmed.aah3438.

Mishra, Priyadarsee, Abhishek Kumar, Prabhudutta Mamidi, Sameer Kumar, Itishree Basantray, Tanuja Saswat, Indrani Das, et al., 2016. "Inhibition of Chikungunya Virus Replication by 1-((2-Methylbenzimidazol-1-Yl) Methyl)-2-Oxo-Indolin-3-Ylidene) Amino) Thiourea(MBZM-N-IBT)." *Scientific Reports* 6 (February): 20122.

Mounce, Bryan C., Teresa Cesaro, Lucia Carrau, Thomas Vallet, and Marco Vignuzzi. 2017. "Curcumin Inhibits Zika and Chikungunya Virus

Infection by Inhibiting Cell Binding." *Antiviral Research* 142 (June): 148–57. https://doi.org/10.1016/j.antiviral.2017.03.014.

Narwal, Manju, Harvijay Singh, Shivendra Pratap, Anjali Malik, Richard J. Kuhn, Pravindra Kumar, and Shailly Tomar. 2018. "Crystal Structure of Chikungunya Virus nsP2 Cysteine Protease Reveals a Putative Flexible Loop Blocking Its Active Site." *International Journal of Biological Macromolecules* 116 (September): 451–62. https://doi.org/10.1016/j.ijbiomac.2018.05.007.

Parashar, Deepti, and Sarah Cherian. 2014. "Antiviral Perspectives for Chikungunya Virus." *BioMed Research International* 2014 (May): 631642. https://doi.org/10.1155/2014/631642.

Pérez-Pérez, María-Jesús, Leen Delang, Lisa F. P. Ng, and Eva-María Priego. 2019. "Chikungunya Virus Drug Discovery: Still a Long Way to Go?" *Expert Opinion on Drug Discovery*. https://doi.org/10.1080/17460441.2019.1629413.

Pratyush Kumar Das, Andres Merits, Aleksei lulla (2014). Functional cross-talk between distant domains of chikungunya virus non-structural protein 2 is decisive for its RNA-modulating activity. *The Journal of biological chemistry*, 289(9), 5635–5653. https:// doi.org/10.1074/jbc.M113.503433.

Rawlings, Neil D., Alan J. Barrett, Paul D. Thomas, Xiaosong Huang, Alex Bateman, and Robert D. Finn. 2018. "The MEROPS Database of Proteolytic Enzymes, Their Substrates and Inhibitors in 2017 and a Comparison with Peptidases in the PANTHER Database." *Nucleic Acids Research* 46 (D1): D624–32.

Roques, Pierre, Simon-Djamel Thiberville, Laurence Dupuis-Maguiraga, Fok-Moon Lum, Karine Labadie, Frédéric Martinon, Gabriel Gras, et al., 2018. "Paradoxical Effect of Chloroquine Treatment in Enhancing Chikungunya Virus Infection." *Viruses* 10 (5). https://doi.org/10.3390/v10050268.

Rupp, Jonathan C., Kevin J. Sokoloski, Natasha N. Gebhart, and Richard W. Hardy. 2015. "Alphavirus RNA Synthesis and Non-Structural Protein Functions." *Journal of General Virology*. 96 (9): 2483–2500. https://doi.org/10.1099/jgv.0.000249.

Russo, Andrew T., Mark A. White, and Stanley J. Watowich. 2006. "The Crystal Structure of the Venezuelan Equine Encephalitis Alphavirus nsP2 Protease." *Structure* 14 (9): 1449–58. https://doi.org/ 10.1016/ j.str.2006.07.010.

Sá, Priscilla Karen de Oliveira, Michaela de Miranda Nunes, Ingrid Ramalho Leite, Maria das Graças Loureiro das Chagas Campelo, Cláudia Ferreira Ribeiro Leão, Joelma Rodrigues de Souza, Lúcio Roberto Castellano, and Ana Isabel Vieira Fernandes. 2017. "Chikungunya Virus Infection with Severe Neurologic Manifestations: Report of Four Fatal Cases." *Revista Da Sociedade Brasileira de Medicina Tropical* 50 (2): 265–68. https://doi.org/10.1590/0037-8682-0375-2016. [*Journal of the Brazilian Society of Tropical Medicine*]

Schnierle, Barbara S. 2019. "Cellular Attachment and Entry Factors for Chikungunya Virus." *Viruses* 11 (11). https://doi.org/10.3390/v111 11078.

Schwartz, Olivier, and Matthew L. Albert. 2010. "Biology and Pathogenesis of Chikungunya Virus." *Nature Reviews Microbiology*. https://doi.org/ 10.1038/nrmicro2368.

Silva-Júnior, Edeildo F. da, Edeildo F. da Silva-Júnior, Giovanni O. Leoncini, Érica E. S. Rodrigues, Thiago M. Aquino, and João X. Araújo-Júnior. 2017. "The Medicinal Chemistry of Chikungunya Virus." *Bioorganic & Medicinal Chemistry.* https://doi.org/10. 1016/j.bmc. 2017.06.049.

Silva, Laurie A., and Terence S. Dermody. 2017. "Chikungunya Virus: Epidemiology, Replication, Disease Mechanisms, and Prospective Intervention Strategies." *The Journal of Clinical Investigation* 127 (3): 737–49. https://doi.org/10.1172/jci84417

Solignat, Maxime, Bernard Gay, Stephen Higgs, Laurence Briant, and Christian Devaux. 2009. "Replication Cycle of Chikungunya: A Re-Emerging Arbovirus." *Virology* 393 (2): 183–97. https://doi.org/ 10.1016/j.virol.2009.07.024.

Soumendranath, Bhakat and Mahmoud E. S. Soliman. 2015. "Chikungunya Virus (CHIKV) Inhibitors from Natural Sources: A Medicinal

Chemistry Perspective." *Journal of Natural Medicines* 69 (4): 451–62. https://doi.org/10.1007/s11418-015-0910-z.

Story, Randall M., Irene T. Weber, and Thomas A. Steitz. 1992. "Erratum: The Structure of the E. Colt recA Protein Monomer and Polymer." *Nature*. https://doi.org/10.1038/355567a0.

Strauss, J. H., and E. G. Strauss. 1994. "The Alphaviruses: Gene Expression, Replication, and Evolution." *Microbiological Reviews* 58 (3): 491–562.

Subudhi, Bharat Bhusan, Soma Chattopadhyay, Priyadarsee Mishra, and Abhishek Kumar. 2018. "Current Strategies for Inhibition of Chikungunya Infection." *Viruses* 10 (5). https://doi.org/10. 3390/v10050235.

Tang, Bor Luen. 2012. "The Cell Biology of Chikungunya Virus Infection." *Cellular Microbiology*. https://doi.org/10.1111/j.1462-5822.2012.01825.x.

Wada, Yuji, Yasuko Orba, Michihito Sasaki, Shintaro Kobayashi, Michael J. Carr, Haruaki Nobori, Akihiko Sato, William W. Hall, and Hirofumi Sawa. 2017. "Discovery of a Novel Antiviral Agent Targeting the Nonstructural Protein 4 (nsP4) of Chikungunya Virus." *Virology* 505 (May): 102–12. https://doi.org/10.1016/j.virol.2017.02.014.

Wang, Yu-Ming, Jeng-Wei Lu, Chang-Chi Lin, Yuan-Fan Chin, Tzong-Yuan Wu, Liang-In Lin, Zheng-Zong Lai, Szu-Cheng Kuo, and Yi-Jung Ho. 2016. "Antiviral Activities of Niclosamide and Nitazoxanide against Chikungunya Virus Entry and Transmission." *Antiviral Research* 135 (November): 81–90. https://doi.org/10.1016/j.antiviral.2016.10.003.

Weaver, Scott C., and Marc Lecuit. 2015. "Chikungunya Virus and the Global Spread of a Mosquito-Borne Disease." *New England Journal of Medicine*. https://doi.org/10.1056/nejmra1406035.

Weber, Christopher, Katja Sliva, Christine von Rhein, Beate M. Kümmerer, and Barbara S. Schnierle. 2015. "The Green Tea Catechin, Epigallocatechin Gallate Inhibits Chikungunya Virus Infection." *Antiviral Research* 113 (January): 1–3. https://doi.org/10.1016/j.antiviral.2014.11.001.

Yiu-Wing Kam, Wendy W. L. Lee, Diane Simarmata, Sumitro Harjanto, Terk-Shin Teng, Hugues Tolou, Angela Chow, Raymond T. P. Lin, Yee-Sin Leo, Laurent Rénia, and Lisa F. P. Nga, 2012, "Longitudinal analysis of the human antibody response to Chikungunya virus infection: implications for serodiagnosis and vaccine development." *J Virol.* 2012;86(23):13005-13015. doi:10.1128/JVI.01780-12.

Zhang, Sixue, Atefeh Garzan, Nicole Haese, Robert Bostwick, Yohanka Martinez-Gzegozewska, Lynn Rasmussen, Daniel N. Streblow, et al., 2021. "Pyrimidone Inhibitors Targeting Chikungunya Virus nsP3 Macrodomain by Fragment-Based Drug Design." *PloS One* 16 (1): e0245013.

INDEX

H

I

J

L

M

N

V

W